Infectious Disease Pearls

Infectious Disease Pearls

BURKE A. CUNHA, MD
Chief, Infectious Disease Division
Winthrop-University Hospital
Mineola, New York
Professor of Medicine
State University of New York
 School of Medicine
Stony Brook, New York

Series Editors

STEVEN A. SAHN, MD
Professor of Medicine and Director
Division of Pulmonary and
 Critical Care Medicine
Medical University of South Carolina
Charleston, South Carolina

JOHN E. HEFFNER, MD
Professor and Vice Chairman
Department of Medicine
Medical University of South Carolina
Charleston, South Carolina

HANLEY & BELFUS, INC. / Philadelphia

Publisher: HANLEY & BELFUS, INC.
                Medical Publishers
                210 S. 13th Street
                Philadelphia, PA 19107
                (215) 546-7293, 800-962-1892
                FAX (215) 790-9330
                Website: http://www.hanleyandbelfus.com

Library of Congress Cataloging-in-Publication Data

Infectious disease pearls / edited by Burke A. Cunha.
        p.   cm. — (The Pearls Series®)
    Includes bibliographical references and index.
    ISBN 1-56053-203-3 (alk. paper)
    1. Communicable diseases—Diagnosis—Case studies.   I. Cunha,
Burke A.   II. Series
    [DNLM: 1. Communicable Diseases case studies.   WC 100 I4028 1999]
RC113.3.I54   1999
616.9′049—dc21
DNLM/DLC   98-40802
for Library of Congress   CIP

INFECTIOUS DISEASE PEARLS   ISBN 1-56053-203-3

Last digit is the print number: 9 8 7 6 5 4 3 2 1

CONTENTS

CONTRIBUTORS

Burke A. Cunha, MD   *Patients 49–64*
Chief, Infectious Disease Division,
Winthrop-University Hospital, Mineola;
Professor of Medicine,
State University of New York School of Medicine,
Stony Brook, New York

M. Vanessa Gill, MD   *Patients 65–77*
Director of Infectious Diseases,
Peebles Hospital,
Tortola, British West Indies

Diane H. Johnson, MD   *Patients 1–20*
Assistant Director, Infectious Disease Division,
Winthrop-University Hospital, Mineola;
Assistant Professor of Medicine,
State University of New York School of Medicine,
Stony Brook, New York

Natalie C. Klein, MD, PhD   *Patients 21–40*
Associate Director, Infectious Disease Division,
Winthrop-University Hospital, Mineola;
Assistant Professor of Medicine,
State University of New York School of Medicine,
Stony Brook, New York

Antonio M. Ortega, MD   *Patients 78–85*
Infectious Disease Private Practice,
El Paso, Texas

Kevin W. Shea, MD   *Patients 41–48*
Director of Infectious Diseases,
Carolinas Hospital System,
Florence, South Carolina

FOREWORD

The Pearls Series® presents challenging clinical problems in a style that provides engaging reading as well as state-of-the-art information. Each case focuses on the puzzle created by the patient's clinical manifestations; the clinician, with careful deliberation, inserts diagnostic clues until a unifying diagnostic pattern emerges. Few topics are so well adapted to the detective work of clinical medicine than the care of patients with infectious diseases.

Infectious Disease Pearls follows The Pearls Series® approach by describing 85 patients with a broad array of infectious conditions in a manner that challenges clinicians to identify the important aspects and reach a working diagnosis and plan for further evaluation or therapeutic care. The discussion that follows each presentation reviews the patient's general disorder and then focuses on unique characteristics. So as not to lose sight of our interest in the individual, the discussion closes with the clinical outcome of the patient. Finally, points of diagnosis and care that are especially important—"cutting edge"—or not widely recognized are captured and listed as "Clinical Pearls."

Student readers beginning their medical careers, residents in training, and experienced clinicians honing their skills will find something of value in each of the patient presentations.

We greatly appreciate the efforts of Dr. Burke A. Cunha in making *Infectious Disease Pearls* the 11th book in The Pearls Series®. We hope that the information provided will assist clinicians in translating the Clinical Pearls into astute bedside care for patients with infectious disorders.

STEVEN A. SAHN, MD
JOHN E. HEFFNER, MD

PREFACE

The value of The Pearls Series® is its distillation of the clinical and educational essence of patient cases into capsular form. Infectious diseases is a discipline that particularly lends itself to this format because, as in internal medicine, the focus is on evaluating differential diagnostic possibilities. In fact, the main difficulty in the field of infectious diseases is not determining appropriate treatment, but ascertaining the correct clinical diagnosis.

We do not have invasive tests and procedures, as are found in cardiology, pulmonary and critical care medicine, and gastroenterology, for example. We cannot employ cybernetic models for problem solving, like endocrinologists. We do not rely on computation, as in nephrology, or physical diagnosis, as in noninvasive cardiology and neurology, or specific laboratory tests, as in hematology/oncology.

In the field of infectious diseases, we rely on cognitive analytical skills to solve our diagnostic problems.

It has been said that infectious diseases resemble acute rheumatologic diseases, and rheumatologic disorders resemble acute infectious diseases. Infectious disease clinicians arrive at a working differential diagnosis in a manner similar to that of rheumatologists: pattern association based on historical context. Therefore, the most important part of each case in *Infectious Disease Pearls* is the discussion, based on the initial history and admission laboratory tests, where diagnostic considerations are emphasized.

This book is intended to challenge the primary care provider, inform the internist, and educate the student. I hope it fulfills its purpose.

BURKE A. CUNHA, MD
EDITOR

Dedication

To our fine sons,
Zac and Chet.

B.A.C.

PATIENT 1

A 50-year-old woman with watery diarrhea receiving ampicillin for a urinary tract infection

A 50-year-old woman presents to the office with a 3-day history of watery diarrhea accompanied by crampy abdominal pain. She is having 10–12 bowel movements in a 24-hour period and is awakened from sleep to use the bathroom. She has a low-grade fever, but denies nausea, vomiting, and blood in the stool. Two weeks ago she was treated with a course of ampicillin for an *Escherichia coli* infection of the urinary tract.

Physical Examination: Temperature 38°; pulse 92; respiration 12; blood pressure 122/80. General: healthy appearance. HEENT: dry mucous membranes. Cardiac: normal. Chest: clear. Abdomen: soft; diffuse, mild tenderness in the right and left lower quadrants; bowel sounds hyperactive. Rectal: trace heme-positive stool. Extremities: no edema. Skin: no rashes or lesions.

Laboratory Findings: WBC 16,200/μl with 90% neutrophils, 8% bands, 2% lymphocytes. BUN 40 mg/dl; creatinine 1.2 mg/dl. Flexible sigmoidoscopy: see figure.

Question: What is the probable diagnosis?

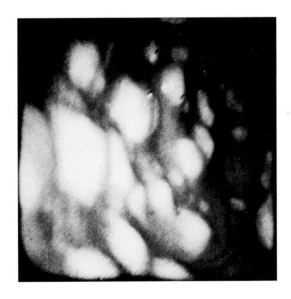

Diagnosis: *Clostridium difficile*-associated pseudomembranous colitis

Discussion: *Clostridium difficile* is a spore-forming, anaerobic, gram-positive rod that is a cause of pseudomembranous colitis. Persons at risk for developing this entity include hospitalized patients and persons who have received antibiotics. *C. difficile*-associated pseudomembranous colitis can occur up to 2 months after offending antibiotics have been discontinued. Almost all antibiotics have been implicated in the development of *C. difficile* colitis, but the incidence appears to be higher after therapy with **clindamycin, ampicillin, and the cephalosporins.** *C. difficile* has been isolated from the hands of hospital staff, and nosocomial spread of this organism is responsible for some cases of disease.

The disorder occurs when intestinal flora are altered by the antimicrobial agent, spores germinate, and the organism proliferates. Toxigenic strains of *C. difficile* coproduce two toxins, A and B, that are responsible for clinical illness. Disease severity ranges from a mild diarrheal illness to fulminant disease. Signs and symptoms include watery or mucoid diarrhea (stools may be bloody), crampy abdominal pain, fevers, abdominal tenderness, and leukocytosis. Rarely, patients present with an acute abdomen: perforation and toxic megacolon have occurred.

The gold standard for the diagnosis of *C. difficile*-associated diarrhea is the **tissue culture cytotoxin assay**, which detects toxin B in the stool. It is a highly specific test; however, results are not available for at least 18 hours, and the laboratory must have tissue culture capability. Enzyme immunoassay (EIA) for the presence of toxins A and B is more easily and quickly performed and has a reasonable level of sensitivity and specificity. Latex agglutination testing and directly culturing *C. difficile* from the stool are alternative methods, but both have high false-positive rates because they detect nontoxin-producing strains of the bacteria.

The presence of **pseudomembranes** on sigmoidoscopy or colonoscopy is diagnostic for *C. difficile* colitis. However, this testing is invasive and expensive. Pseudomembranes are occasionally isolated to the ascending or transverse colon; these lesions would be missed if only sigmoidoscopy was performed.

Therapy for *C. difficile* colitis consists of discontinuing the offending antibiotic, if possible, and administering oral **metronidazole** or **vancomycin.** In general, antiperistaltic agents should be avoided. Severely ill patients or patients unable to take oral agents should be treated with intravenous metronidazole.

The present patient's stool was positive for *C. difficile* toxin B, and pseudomembranous plaques were evident in the sigmoid colon (see figure). She was given a course of oral metronidazole, and her diarrhea gradually improved over several days. She completed a 1-week course of therapy and had no further recurrence of her symptoms.

Clinical Pearls

1. *C. difficile*-associated pseudomembranous colitis can occur up to 2 months after antibiotics have been discontinued.

2. Although β-lactams and clindamycin are most frequently implicated, any antimicrobial can cause *C. difficile* colitis.

3. The stool cytotoxicity assay for toxin B is the gold standard in the diagnosis of *C. difficile*-associated diarrhea.

REFERENCES
1. Bartlett JG: Antibiotic-associated diarrhea. Clin Infect Dis 1992; 15:573–581.
2. Fekety R, Shah AB: Diagnosis and treatment of *C. difficile* colitis. JAMA 1993; 269:71–75.
3. Mitty RD, Lamont JT: *Clostridium difficile* diarrhea: Pathogenesis, epidemiology, and treatment. Gastroenterol 1994; 2:61–69.

PATIENT 2

A 19-year-old man with dysuria, frequent urination, and purulent urethral discharge

A 19-year-old college student presents to the student health service complaining of dysuria, frequent urination, and a purulent urethral discharge. He denies fever, rash, sore throat, and joint pains. He is sexually active with one partner and regularly uses condoms, with one exception 2 weeks previously when he visited a prostitute during an alcohol binge. He takes no medications and is not allergic to any antibiotics.

Physical Examination: Temperature 37.1°; pulse 76. General: anxious-appearing. HEENT: unremarkable. Chest: clear. Cardiac: normal S_1S_2, no murmurs. Abdomen: soft, nontender, no masses or organomegaly. Extremities: no joint swelling. Skin: no rashes or lesions. Genitourinary: testes descended bilaterally, no masses, no tenderness, no penile lesions; copious purulent urethral discharge. Lymph nodes: no inguinal adenopathy.

Laboratory Examination: Urethral exudate Gram stain: 20 WBC/oil immersion field; some intracellular gram-negative diplococci. Urethral culture: positive for *Neisseria gonorrhoeae* (see figure). Venereal Disease Research Laboratory test: nonreactive. Fluorescent treponemal antibody: negative.

Question: What is the likely diagnosis?

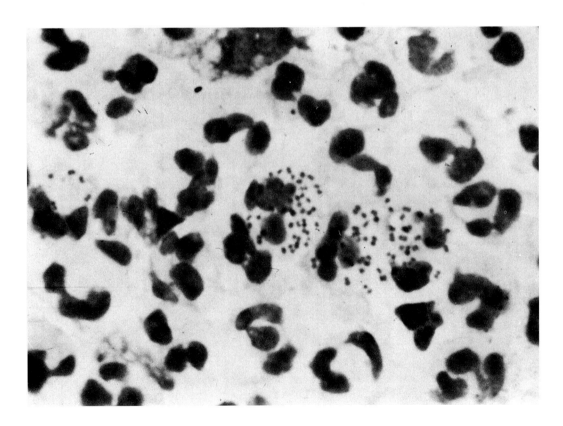

Diagnosis: Gonorrhea

Discussion: Gonorrhea is an infection of the epithelial cells of the urethra, cervix, pharynx, rectum, or eyes caused by the gram-negative coccus *N. gonorrhoeae*. Humans are the only natural hosts for this infection, which is spread through close sexual contact, usually with individuals who are asymptomatic or who have chosen to ignore their symptoms.

In men, the usual incubation period of gonococcal urethritis is approximately 1 week. Initial symptoms include dysuria, frequent urination, and a profuse, purulent urethral discharge. Additionally, the urinary meatus may be erythematous. Untreated persons are at risk for developing epididymitis, prostatitis, and local complications such as dorsal lymphangitis or thrombophlebitis of the penis, periurethral abscesses or fistulas, and inguinal lymphadenitis.

Gonorrhea in women may be more subtle. Symptoms of dysuria and frequent urination may be present, but often are attributed to cystitis. Vaginal discharge is common, and on pelvic examination the cervix appears reddened and friable. Endometritis and salpingitis are not uncommon and present with abdominal pain and abnormal menstrual bleeding. Other complications include extension of infection to the pelvis or into the upper abdomen, causing perihepatitis (Fitz-Hugh-Curtis syndrome). The Bartholin's glands and Skene's ducts may be involved, as well.

A Gram stain of urethral exudate or endocervical pus that reveals leukocytes containing **gram-negative diplococci** is diagnostic of gonococcal infection; however, the sensitivity of the Gram stain only approaches 60% in women. Culture always should be performed in women *and* men with an equivocal or negative Gram stain. Selective media such as modified Thayer Martin or New York City agar is required, and the specimen must be incubated at 36° in an atmosphere containing 3–10% CO_2. Serologic testing for gonorrhea is not clinically useful, but serologic testing for syphilis should be performed on all persons suspected of having a sexually transmitted disease.

Therapy of uncomplicated endocervical or urethral infection is one dose of **ceftriaxone**, 125 mg intramuscularly. Alternatively, one-dose therapy with oral cefixime, ciprofloxacin, ofloxacin or intramuscular spectinomycin can be used. Because penicillin- and tetracycline-resistant strains of *N. gonorrhoeae* are widespread, these agents should not be used. All patients with gonorrhea should be treated simultaneously for **chlamydial infection,** which often is present in patients with gonorrhea.

The present patient's urethral culture confirmed the diagnosis of gonorrhea. Gram stain of urethral secretions showed numerous polymorphonuclear leukocytes and intracellular gram-negative diplococci (see figure). He was given an intramuscular dose of ceftriaxone and a 7-day course of oral doxycycline to treat a possible chlamydial infection. The patient never returned for a routine follow-up visit; however, he presented 6 months later with similar symptoms and again was diagnosed with gonorrhea. He again admitted to episodes of unprotected intercourse.

Clinical Pearls

1. Gonorrhea often is spread by asymptomatic carriers.
2. A Gram stain of urethral or endocervical exudate that reveals leukocytes containing gram-negative diplococci is diagnostic for gonorrhea.
3. All patients with gonorrhea should be treated simultaneously for infection with *Chlamydia trachomatis.*

REFERENCES
1. Dallabetta G, Hook EW III: Gonococcal infections. Infect Dis Clin North Am 1987; 1:25–54.
2. Judson FN: Gonorrhea. Med Clin North Am 1990; 74:1353–1366.
3. Moy JG, Clasen ME: The patient with gonococcal infection. Prim Care 1990; 17:59–83.
4. Handsfield HH: Recent developments in STDs. I. Bacterial diseases. Hosp Pract (Off Ed) 1991; 26:47–56.
5. Abramowicz M (ed): Drugs for sexually transmitted diseases. Med Lett Drugs Ther 1994; 36(913):1–6.

PATIENT 3

A 3-year-old child with fever and nuchal rigidity

A 3-year-old girl presents to the emergency department with fever to 39.8°C and lethargy. Her mother states she has no prior medical problems, but has been ill with a cold for several days. Immunization history is unknown, but the mother states "she has missed a few shots."

Physical Examination: Temperature 39.8°; pulse 130; respirations 22. General: lethargic, but arousable. Cardiac: tachycardic, no murmurs. HEENT: pharynx and tympanic membranes mildly injected; minimal, clear nasal discharge. Chest: clear. Abdomen: soft, nontender, bowel sounds present, no masses. Extremities: no edema. Skin: no rashes. Neurologic: nuchal rigidity present, positive Kernig and Brudzinski signs, no focal deficits.

Laboratory Findings: WBC 15,600/μl with 90% neutrophils, 6% bands, 4% lymphocytes. Cerebrospinal fluid (CSF): opening pressure 300 mmHg; WBC 15,000/μl with 98% neutrophils, 2% lymphocytes; protein 160 mg/dl; glucose 15 mg/dl. CSF Gram stain: moderate WBCs and small, gram-negative rods (see figure).

Question: What diagnosis is most probable, and how would you proceed?

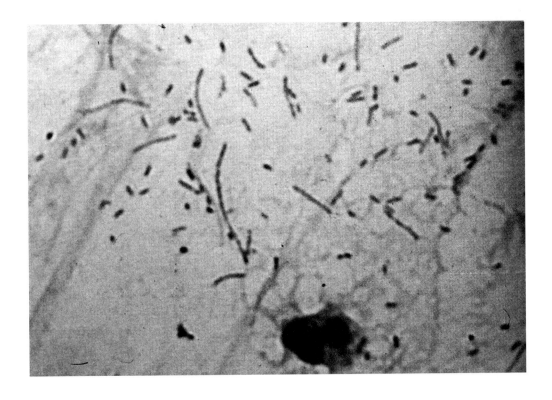

Diagnosis: *Haemophilus influenzae* meningitis

Discussion: *Haemophilus influenzae* meningitis is the most common cause of meningitis in young children, although there has been a marked decrease in the number of infections caused by this pathogen since the release of *Haemophilus influenzae* type B (HiB) vaccine. Occasionally, *H. influenzae* meningitis is encountered in an adult; an underlying condition such as diabetes or alcoholism or an anatomic defect such as a CSF leak usually is present in these cases.

Upper respiratory tract infections or otitis media may precede meningeal infection. The clinical picture—with fever, headache, lethargy, and stiff neck—is similar to that of meningitis caused by other bacterial agents. Seizures and cranial nerve palsies may be encountered; rarely, a petechial rash is found. Kernig's and Brudzinski's signs may be absent in very young children. Laboratory findings also are similar to those found in other forms of purulent meningitis, with an elevated CSF opening pressure and a CSF leukocytosis usually featuring ≥ 1000 cells/μl and a neutrophilic predominance. CSF chemistries reveal elevated protein and depressed glucose levels. Gram stain of the spinal fluid is positive in approximately 75% of untreated patients with *H. influenzae* appearing as a pleomorphic gram-negative rod. Occasionally, the organism stains heavily at the poles and is confused with pneumococci. Cultures of CSF are positive in about 75% of cases. Latex agglutination testing or counterimmunoelectrophoresis may be helpful in patients previously treated with antibiotics.

Some strains of *H. influenzae* produce β-lactamases. This is an important consideration when choosing an antimicrobial drug. A **third-generation cephalosporin** is the drug of choice in the treatment of *H. influenzae* meningitis. Alternatively, a combination of ampicillin and chloramphenicol can be used. Corticosteroids administered early along with antibiotics probably are useful in preventing sequelae such as hearing loss in *H. influenzae* meningitis. Close contacts of patients with *H. influenzae* meningitis should receive chemoprophylaxis with rifampin administered for 4 doses. The index case should be given rifampin as well, since some antibiotics may not eliminate nasopharyngeal colonization with the organism.

The present patient was treated with ceftriaxone and corticosteroids over a 10-day course. The CSF Gram stain demonstrated *H. influenzae,* which subsequently grew on culture. The patient's parents and younger siblings all received a 2-day course of rifampin. The patient was discharged home and continues to do well.

Clinical Pearls

1. The incidence of *H. influenzae* meningitis has been decreasing since the release of the *H. influenzae* type B vaccine.

2. *H. influenzae* meningitis often is preceded by upper respiratory tract infections or otitis media.

3. Corticosteroids administered early in children with *H. influenzae* meningitis appear to decrease morbidity.

4. Both close contacts and the index case should receive chemoprophylaxis with rifampin to eradicate nasopharyngeal carriage.

REFERENCES

1. Kennedy WA, Hoyt MT, McCracken GH: The role of corticosteroid therapy in children with pneumococcal meningitis. Am J Dis Child 1991; 145:1374–1378.
2. Geiman BJ, Smith AL: Dexamethasone and bacterial meningitis: A meta-analysis of randomized controlled trials. West J Med 1992; 157:27–31.
3. McCracken GH Jr: Current management of bacterial meningitis in infants and children. Pediatr Infect Dis J 1992; 11:169–174.
4. Turkel AR, Scheld WM: Acute meningitis. *In* Mandell GL, Bennett JE, Dolin R (eds): Principles and Practice of Infectious Diseases. 4th ed. New York, Churchill Livingstone, 1995, pp 831–864.

PATIENT 4

A 21-year-old woman with pneumonia and acute myelogenous leukemia

A 21-year-old woman with acute myelogenous leukemia is hospitalized for a febrile leukopenic episode. She is status post chemotherapy and had been placed on broad-spectrum antibiotic coverage that resulted in rapid defervescence and clinical improvement. Subsequently, all cultures drawn on admission are negative. A few days later, she develops fever to 39.6°C accompanied by increasing dyspnea and pleuritic chest pain. Medications are vancomycin, ceftazidime, gentamicin, acetominophen, and granulocyte colony–stimulating factor. She has no known medication allergies.

Physical Examination: Temperature 39.6°; pulse 130; respirations 22; blood pressure 90/58. General: ill-appearing. HEENT: no abnormalities. Chest: bibasilar crackles. Cardiac: tachycardic, normal S_1S_2, grade II/VI systolic murmur. Abdomen: soft, nontender; normal bowel sounds. Extremities: trace pedal edema. Skin: no rashes or lesions.

Laboratory Findings: Hct 25%; WBC 100/μl (unable to perform differential); platelets 60,000/μl. Creatinine 1.3 mg/dl. Blood cultures: negative. Sputum Gram stain: no cells or organisms. Sputum KOH: few fungal elements, with septate hyphae branching at acute angles. Chest radiograph: vague infiltrate in right lower lobe.

Question: What complication of pneumonia has occurred?

Diagnosis: Pulmonary aspergillosis

Discussion: *Aspergillus* species are molds that are encountered worldwide, most commonly in soil, hay, grain, and decaying vegetation. The airborne spores of this mold cause disease after being inhaled or by invasion through skin portals. **Immunocompromised hosts,** such as transplant patients, granulocytopenic patients, and those in the late stages of acquired immunodeficiency disease, are at highest risk for serious infection with the organism.

Patients with prolonged neutropenia are susceptible to developing pulmonary infection with *Aspergillus* species. Pneumonia most often is caused by *A. fumigatus,* although *A. flavus* and other species also have been described. Infection in these cases is likely due to inhalation of spores, but gastrointestinal or previous pulmonary colonization may play a role in disease.

The most common clinical manifestation of *Aspergillus* pneumonia is a **persistently elevated temperature.** Pulmonary complaints may be absent, or consist of dyspnea, pleuritic chest pain, or hemoptysis. Hypoxemia frequently is seen. Generally, radiographic findings are either those of bronchopneumonia or multiple patchy infiltrates. Nodular densities, an interstitial pattern, or a cavitary lesion also may be present. Since *Aspergillus* species can invade blood vessels, it may be difficult to interpret whether the radiographic findings represent infiltrate or pulmonary infarction. In patients who are profoundly neutropenic, infiltrates may be vague or absent.

The diagnosis of *Aspergillus* pneumonia can be difficult. In hosts who are at risk for the development of invasive disease—such as granulocytopenic patients or those receiving immunosuppressive therapy—the isolation of *Aspergillus* from respiratory secretions has been strongly correlated with invasive pulmonary aspergillosis. However, a negative sputum Grain stain or culture does not rule out the presence of disease. Bronchoalveolar lavage (BAL) specimens increase diagnostic yield when sputum studies are negative, but again, a negative BAL does not preclude the presence of invasive disease. If the diagnosis remains in question or if the patient is not responding to therapy, then open lung biopsy should be employed to check for *Aspergillus* invasion of lung tissue (see figure at right). Computed tomography or magnetic resonance imaging may be an important adjunct in diagnosis since early cavitation is suggestive of pulmonary aspergillosis.

Aspergillus pneumonia in the immunocompromised host has a poor prognosis because typically there is dissemination of the fungus and abscess formation in the central nervous system, eye, gastrointestinal and genitourinary tracts, and liver. Cutaneous nodules may present on the skin of patients with disseminated disease.

Successful treatment of pulmonary aspergillosis depends on several factors, including early recognition of the disease, reversal of the granulocytopenia, and, if possible, discontinuation of immunosuppression.

Amphotericin B remains the mainstay of treatment for invasive pulmonary aspergillosis, usually at doses of 1.0–1.5 mg/kg/day. Lipid formulations of amphotericin B can be used in patients who are intolerant to amphotericin B. Itraconazole is active against *Aspergillus* as well, but is generally used in patients who are clinically stable.

The present patient was begun empirically on amphotericin B. She subsequently developed nodular skin lesions which, when biopsied, revealed the same septate branching hyphae. Despite intensive therapy, the patient died a few days later.

Clinical Pearls

1. In granulocytopenic patients, invasive pulmonary aspergillosis may present only with an elevated temperature; infiltrates may be vague or nonexistent.

2. The presence of septate hyphae branching at acute angles in the sputum suggests aspergillosis in the immunocompromised patient and strongly correlates with the presence of invasive disease.

3. Metastatic abscess formation in the brain, liver, and kidneys is common in aspergillosis in the compromised host.

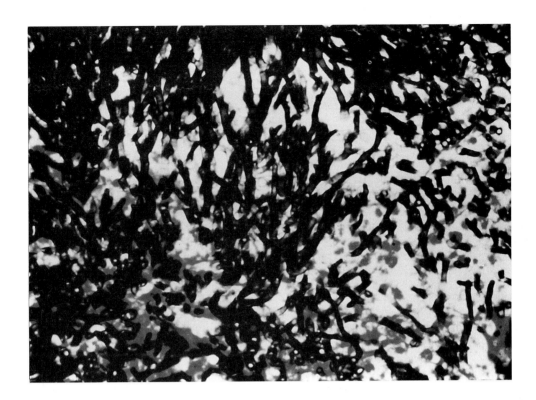

REFERENCES

1. Fisher BD, Armstrong D, Yu B, et al: Invasive aspergillosis: Progress in early diagnosis and treatment. Am J Med 1981; 71:571–577.
2. Anaissie E, Bodey GP, Kantarjian H, et al: New spectrum of fungal infections in patients with cancer. Rev Infect Dis 1989; 11:369–378.
3. Walsh TJ, Hiemenz JW, Anaissie E: Recent progress in current problems in treatment of invasive fungal infections in neutropenic patients. Infect Dis Clin North Am 1996; 10:365–400.

PATIENT 5

A 70-year-old woman with bilateral, rapidly progressing pneumonia during an influenza outbreak

A 70-year-old woman presents to the emergency department with fever and severe dyspnea. Several days before, while at a New Year's Eve party, she experienced abrupt onset of fever, chills, headache, myalgia, and sore throat. She also complains of a nonproductive cough that has progressively worsened. Past medical history includes hypertension and coronary artery disease. The patient has no known drug allergies.

Physical Examination: Temperature 38.8°; pulse 110, respirations 36; blood pressure 160/84. General: ill-appearing, moderate respiratory distress. HEENT: mild conjunctival and pharyngeal injection. Neck: supple, no adenopathy. Cardiac: tachycardic, I/VI systolic ejection murmur. Chest: bilateral, diffuse crackles; expiratory wheezes. Abdomen: soft, nontender, no organomegaly. Extremities: peripheral cyanosis. Skin: diaphoretic, mottled.

Laboratory Findings: WBC 12, 800/μl with 68% neutrophils, 2% bands, 30% lymphocytes. BUN 48 mg/dl; creatinine 1.6 mg/dl. Throat culture and sensitivity: normal. Chest radiograph: bilateral, diffuse, interstitial opacities. Pulse oximetry: 86% O_2 saturation on room air.

Questions: What diagnosis should be considered? How would you treat the patient?

Diagnosis: Primary influenza pneumonia

Discussion: The influenza viruses (A, B, and C) cause upper and lower respiratory disease in the host and usually present as epidemics during the winter months. They are acquired through contact with the respiratory secretions of infected individuals. The onset of influenza is **sudden**. Patients complain of headache, fevers, chills, and myalgias, particularly of the legs and back. Sore throat, which may be severe, also is common. Symptoms relating to the eyes, such as burning, photophobia, and pain on eye motion, also may be present. Physical findings are minimal. The acute illness generally resolves within 1 week, although fatigue may be present for several weeks afterwards.

A major complication of influenza is the development of pneumonia. Primary influenza pneumonia is characterized by the **rapid increase in severity** of pulmonary symptoms. On chest radiograph, diffuse bilateral opacities are found, which may progress to acute respiratory distress syndrome. Hypoxemia is present, often to a severe degree. Sputum production is scant, and cultures yield only normal flora. Individuals at high risk for the development of influenza pneumonia include those with mitral stenosis or chronic underlying pulmonary disease. However, healthy, young adults can be affected as well. In some epidemics, pregnant women have been at high risk for the development of influenza pneumonia.

The diagnosis of primary influenza pneumonia is made clinically (see table next page), and the virus can be isolated or the viral antigens detected in the respiratory secretions. Serologic diagnosis also can be made by demonstrating a fourfold rise in titer between acute and convalescent specimens.

Treatment for influenza pneumonia remains supportive, with administration of supplemental oxygen and hemodynamic support as needed. **Amantidine** and **rimantidine** have been useful in the treatment of uncomplicated influenza when they are begun within 48 hours of symptom onset, but their benefits and the benefits of other antivirals, such as ribavirin, remain unproven in the therapy of influenza pneumonia. Individuals at risk for the development of influenza and its complications should be **vaccinated** on an annual basis, prior to the onset of influenza season.

The present patient presented during the influenza season with classic symptoms of influenza pneumonia. She was initially started on rimantidine. Subsequently, cultures of the pharyngeal washings demonstrated influenza A. The patient completed a 5-day course of rimantidine and was awaiting discharge home after a week of hospitalization when she again developed fever and a cough with purulent sputum. A chest radiograph revealed an opacity in the right middle lobe. The patient was diagnosed with secondary bacterial pneumonia and was treated with antibiotics. She ultimately did well and was discharged home.

Clinical Pearls

1. Patients with primary influenza pneumonia progressively worsen, whereas patients who contract a secondary bacterial pneumonia that complicates influenza generally show clinical improvement before experiencing a relapse of pulmonary symptoms.

2. Primary influenza pneumonia affects young, healthy persons as well as those with cardiorespiratory conditions.

3. The benefit of antiviral medications remains unproven in the treatment of primary influenza pneumonia.

Clinical Presentations of Influenza Pneumonia

	Influenza	Influenza With Bacterial Pneumonia	Influenza Followed By Bacterial Pneumonia
Usual pathogens	Influenza virus	Influenza virus plus *S. aureus*	Influenza virus plus *S. pneumoniae, H. influenzae,* or *S. aureus*
Delay after initial presentation	None	2–3 days following initial improvement	1–3 weeks after initial presentation during convalescence
Symptoms	Severe malaise, restlessness, intermittent dry cough, ± minimal hemoptysis	Ill-appearing, productive cough, sudden deterioration after 2–3 days	Ill-appearing, pneumonia symptoms, productive cough, ± pleuritic chest pain
Signs	No rales, hypoxemic, sternal chest pain, intercostal myalgias mimic pleuritic chest pain	Central cyanosis, hypotension, diffuse rales, very hypoxemic	Fever recurs after becoming afebrile, localized rales, ± decreased breath sounds
WBC count	Normal/decreased	Marked leukocytosis	Leukocytosis
Chest x-ray	Normal/no definite opacities	Multiple opacities, pneumatoceles, pneumothorax, multiple abscesses/ rapid cavitation	Lobar consolidation, no cavitation

Data from Cunha BA, Qadir MT: Viral influenza. Infect Dis Pract 1996; 20:13–14. With permission.

REFERENCES

1. Yinnon AM, Dolin R: Using antivirals to fight influenza in 1991–1992. J Respir Dis 1991; 12:1146.
2. Cunha BA, Qadir MT: Viral influenza. Infect Dis Pract 1996; 20:13–14.
3. Falsey AR: Viral respiratory tract infections in elderly persons. Infect Dis Clin Pract 1996; 5:53–57.

PATIENT 6

A 21-year-old man with fever, tenosynovitis, and 20 pustular lesions on the extremities

A 21-year-old man complains of 3 days of flu-like symptoms with low-grade fever, arthralgias and myalgias. Over the past 24 hours, he has noticed tender, pustular lesions on his hands, feet, arms, and legs. He denies headache, photophobia, meningismus, genital lesions, and penile discharge. Past medical history is significant for genital herpes simplex. There are no known medication allergies.

Physical Examination: Temperature 38.8°; pulse 100; respirations 14; blood pressure 130/72. General: uncomfortable-appearing. HEENT: normal. Chest: clear. Cardiac: regular rate, no murmurs. Abdomen: soft, nontender, no masses, no organomegaly. Genitals: normal, no lesions, no penile discharge. Extremities: swollen, tender, erythematous right wrist. Skin: 20 pustular lesions scattered over upper and lower extremities, including palms and soles (see figure).

Laboratory Findings: WBC 11,200/μl with 80% neutrophils, 9% bands, 5% lymphocytes, 3% monocytes, 3% eosinophils. Electrolytes, BUN, chemistries: normal. Blood cultures: pending. Synovial fluid: WBC 10,000/μl. Gram stain: numerous WBC, no organisms.

Question: What other culture specimen should be obtained?

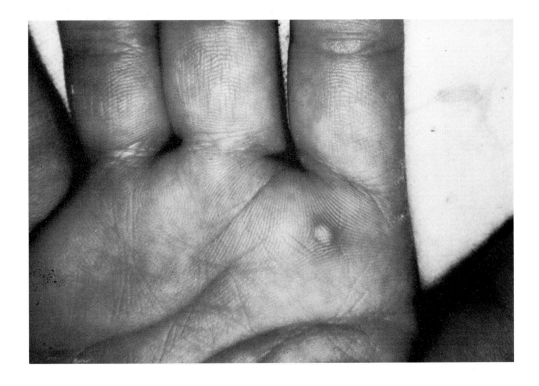

13

Answer: A urethral swab culture

Discussion: Disseminated gonococcal infection is a result of the bacteremic spread of *Neisseria gonorrhoeae*—usually to the skin or articular surfaces, although meningitis, endocarditis, and perihepatitis have occurred, as well. Dissemination occurs in approximately 2% of those infected with gonorrhea; in these cases, overt signs of genital infection may be absent. The most common presentations of disseminated infection are an arthritis-dermatitis syndrome and septic arthritis. Disseminated gonococcal infection is a frequent cause of septic arthritis in young adults.

In the **arthritis-dermatitis syndrome,** patients complain of migratory polyarthralgias with asymmetrical involvement of the wrists, knees, elbows, and hands, low-grade fever, and malaise. Typically, there is objective evidence of tenosynovitis, and a rash may be present peripherally on the extremities (including the palms and soles). The eruption is characterized by a small number (< 40) of discrete papular and pustular lesions that are tender to the touch and may have a hemorrhagic component. Gram stains and cultures of skin lesions usually are negative, but *N. gonorrhoeae* can be isolated from the blood in about 50% of patients. Generally, the synovial fluid is sterile.

Purulent arthritis can occur without prior symptoms of fever, rash, or polyarthritis. Although involvement of the knees, ankles, and wrists is most common, any joint can be affected—including the temporomandibular and sternoclavicular joints. Aspiration of the joint yields pus and, commonly, gonococci are isolated. In 80% of disseminated gonococcal infections, *N. gonorrhoeae* is isolated from the urethra, cervix, rectum, or pharynx.

Treatment of disseminated gonococcal infection includes **repeated joint aspiration** for septic arthritis and **antimicrobial therapy.** Effective agents include intravenous ceftriaxone or an equivalent third-generation cephalosporin. Intramuscular spectinomycin also can be used. After clinical improvement, patients can be switched to an oral agent, such as cefixime or ciprofloxacin, to complete a 10-day course of treatment. Penicillin or tetracycline may be used if the organism is documented as being sensitive.

The present patient was evaluated with a urethral swab culture and two sets of blood cultures, all of which were positive for *N. gonorrhoeae*. The palm lesion (see figure) was a characteristic pustule of disseminated gonorrhea. He was treated with 1 week of intravenous ceftriaxone, and his fevers and skin lesions completely resolved. He was switched to oral ciprofloxacin for the remainder of his course, and on office follow-up several weeks later, he was doing well.

Clinical Pearls

1. Overt signs of genital disease may be absent in disseminated gonococcal infection, but *N. gonorrhoeae* is cultured from a mucosal site in 80% of cases.

2. Unlike immune polyarthritis, which is symmetrical, the arthritis of disseminated gonococcal infection is asymmetrical.

3. Blood cultures generally are positive during the first week of illness.

4. Skin lesions are located distally on the extremities and are few in number.

REFERENCES
1. Keat A: Sexually transmitted arthritis syndrome. Med Clin North Am 1990; 74:1617–1631.
2. Abramowicz M (ed): Drugs for sexually transmitted diseases. The Medical Letter 1994; 36:913.
3. Rich E, Hook EW 3rd, Alarcon GS, et al: Reactive arthritis in patients attending an urban sexually transmitted disease clinic. Arthritis Rheum 1996; 39:1172–1177.

PATIENT 7

A 25-year-old man with a painless, indurated penile ulcer

A 25-year-old man presents to a walk-in medical clinic with a 1-week history of a painless penile lesion. He denies fever, chills, dysuria, and penile discharge. He denies any history of sexually transmitted diseases in the past, but states he has had multiple sexual partners in recent months. The patient notes that his condom use is intermittent. Previous medical history is unremarkable, and there are no known allergies to antibiotics.

Physical Examination: Temperature 36.8°; pulse 62; respirations 12; blood pressure 120/62. General: well-appearing. HEENT: unremarkable. Cardiac: regular rate and rhythm, no extra sounds. Chest: clear bilaterally. Abdomen: soft, nontender, no organ enlargement. Genitalia: testes descended bilaterally, nontender, no masses; indurated, eroded lesion on shaft of penis. Lymph nodes: nontender, bilateral, inguinal adenopathy. Skin: no rashes or lesions.

Laboratory Findings: Venereal Disease Research Laboratory (VDRL) test: 1:64. Flurorescent treponemal antibody, absorbed (FTA-ABS): positive.

Question: What diagnosis is most likely given the patient's clinical and laboratory presentation?

Diagnosis: Primary syphilis

Discussion: Syphilis is a sexually transmitted, systemic disease caused by the spirochete *Treponema pallidum*. It is transmitted by direct contact with an infected individual, as well as by blood transfusions and intrauterine infection. Primary disease commonly manifests as a **chancre**, which is a painless, indurated ulceration at the site of inoculation (see figure below). Chancres generally are located on the penis in men; however, in homosexual men likely locations include the rectum and mouth, and these chancres may not be noticed by the physician. Similarly, primary syphilitic chancres in women typically are found on the labia or vaginal mucosa, but they also may appear—undetected—on the cervix. Multiple chancres can arise, especially in patients with HIV infection. Regional lymphadenopathy, also painless, may accompany the lesion. The chancre resolves spontaneously without treatment in approximately 4 weeks, but the accompanying adenopathy may take several weeks to resolve.

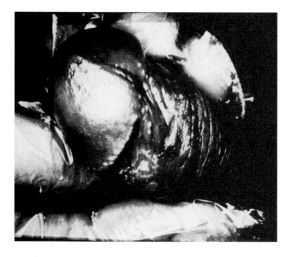

The diagnosis of primary syphilis is made definitively by demonstrating the spirochete with darkfield microscopy or direct fluorescent antibody staining of exudate or tissue from the lesion. Serologic screening for syphilis consists of the nontreponemal tests, such as VDRL, rapid plasmin reagin, and automated reagin. However, these tests can be negative in approximately one third of patients with primary syphilis. The treponemal tests consist of the FTA-ABS and the microhemagglutination-*T. pallidum* (MHA-TP). The FTA-ABS is somewhat more sensitive in primary syphillis, whereas the sensitivity of the MHA-TP is similar to that of the VDRL (80% primary, 100% secondary). The

VDRL can be repeated 2 weeks after the initial negative result in cases where clinical suspicion of primary syphilis is high. False positive nontreponemal tests are thought to account for less than 2% of all positive tests. Common reasons for false positive results include recent illness, autoimmune disease, old age, drug addiction, and other spirochetal diseases such as pinta or yaws. False positive FTA-ABS results are seen with other spirochetal illnesses and in systemic lupus erythematosus; however, in the latter, the pattern of immunofluorescence is atypical. Lyme disease, caused by the spirochete *Borrelia burgdorferi,* yields negative nontreponemal tests, but the FTA-ABS may be positive.

Primary disease is treated with a single dose of 2.4 million units of benzathine penicillin given intramuscularly. In patients with documented penicillin allergy, doxycycline 100 mg twice a day for 2 weeks or tetracycline 500 mg four times a day for 2 weeks can be used, but these regimens are less effective than penicillin injection, and compliance is a problem. Single-dose ceftriaxone should *not* be used at this time for the treatment of syphilis. Syphilis in pregnancy *always* should be treated with penicillin. Pregnant patients who are penicillin-allergic should be appropriately skin tested and desensitized. Persons infected with HIV and primary syphilis are treated with one intramuscular dose of benzathine penicillin. Some experts advocate multiple doses of intramuscular penicillin or augmentation of the initial dose with an additional 1–2 weeks of oral therapy for these patients. Debate continues regarding the utility of an early lumbar puncture in the HIV-infected patient.

Follow-up of the patient with primary syphilis includes repeat serologic testing at 6 and 12 months. If titers increase fourfold or if a titer > 1:32 fails to decline by at least two dilutions, then the patient should be evaluated for reinfection or neurosyphilis and treated appropriately. More frequent serologic testing should occur for HIV-infected individuals, and if a fourfold decrease in titer does not occur within 3 months, a cerebrospinal examination (CSF) should be performed. If the CSF is normal, benzathine penicillin 2.4 million units intramuscularly should be given weekly for three doses.

The present patient was diagnosed with primary syphilis because a chancre is present and a spirochete was isolated from the lesion on darkfield examination. His VDRL was positive at a titer of 1:64, and the FTA was reactive. The patient was given a single intramuscular dose of penicillin. His VDRL declined over the course of a year to 1:2 and, as expected, the FTA remained positive.

Clinical Pearls

1. The chancre of primary syphilis may resemble those of herpes virus infection or chancroid; however, the latter are painful and generally are associated with painful lymphadenopathy.

2. Lyme disease may give a positive FTA-ABS result, but the nontreponemal tests, such as the VDRL, will be negative.

3. Syphilis in pregnancy *always* should be treated with a penicillin regimen, even if desensitization is required.

REFERENCES

1. Centers for Disease Control: Recommendations for diagnosing and treating syphilis in HIV-infected patients. MMWR 1988; 37:600–602, 607–608.
2. Hutchinson CM, Hook EW: Syphilis in adults. Med Clin North Am. 1990; 74:1389–1416.
3. Centers for Disease Control and Prevention: Sexually transmitted disease treatment guidelines. MMWR 1993; 42(RR-14):1–102.
4. Rolfs RT: Treatment of syphilis 1993. Clin Infect Dis 1995; 20 (Suppl 1):S23–S38.
5. Jurado RL: Syphilis serology: A practical approach. Infect Dis Clin Pract 1996; 5:351–358.

PATIENT 8

A 60-year-old woman with fever, headache, and nuchal rigidity

A 60-year-old woman presents to the emergency department with a 1-day history of fever to 38.8°C, shaking chills, frontal headache, and a stiff neck. Upon arrival, she has one episode of vomiting. The patient will not allow the light to be on in the examining room because "it hurts her eyes." She denies ear pain, nasal discharge, and skin rash and states that she has not been ill recently. Past medical history is significant for hypertension. She has no known drug allergies.

Physical Examination: Temperature 39.6°; pulse 122; respirations 12; blood pressure 110/62. General: lethargic and ill-appearing. HEENT: pupils equal, round, reactive to light; no papilledema; tympanic membranes normal; no nasal discharge; pharynx mildly injected. Cardiac: regular rhythm, no murmur. Chest: clear. Abdomen: soft, nontender, no masses, no organomegaly. Extremities: trace pedal edema, no rashes. Neurologic: lethargic, oriented to person and place, positive Kernig's sign, positive Brudzinki's sign.

Laboratory Findings: WBC 31,000/μl with 88% neutrophils, 10% bands, 2% lymphocytes. Serum glucose 110 mg/dl. Cerebrospinal fluid (CSF): opening pressure 250 mm H_2O; WBC 12,500/μl with 95% neutrophils, 4% lymphocytes, 1% other cells; protein 150 mg/dl; glucose 30 mg/dl. Gram stain: moderate WBC, gram-positive diplococci (see figure). Chest radiograph: no opacities.

Questions: What diagnosis should be considered? How should the patient be treated if the diagnosis is confirmed?

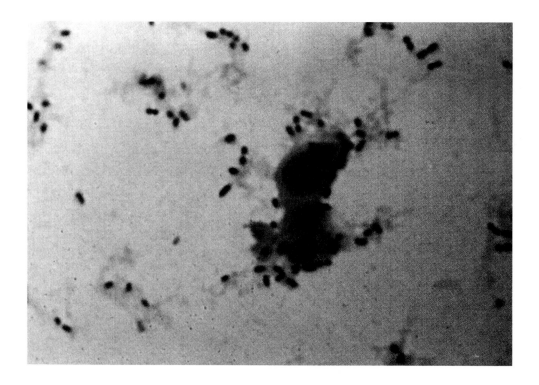

Diagnosis: Pneumococcal meningitis

Discussion: Pneumococci and meningococci are responsible for the majority of cases of adult meningitis. Pneumococcal meningitis can arise as a result of sinusitis or otitis media, as a complication of pneumococcal pneumonia, or in association with a skull fracture and/or CSF leak. It also may develop as a primary disease without an obvious source. Like other pneumococcal processes, it is encountered more frequently in persons with sickle cell disease, hypogammaglobulinemia, multiple myeloma, lymphomas, diabetes mellitus, or alcoholism, and in patients who have undergone a splenectomy.

The clinical presentation of pneumococcal meningitis is similar to infection caused by other pathogens: there are no distinctive clinical features. Headache, fever, chills, photophobia, nuchal rigidity, and possibly Kernig's and Brudzinki's signs may be seen. Cranial nerve palsies, delerium, and coma can occur in pneumococcal meningitis. Evidence of otitis media, pneumonia, sinusitis, or endocarditis may be present. Importantly, signs and symptoms of meningitis may be atypical—especially in very young or elderly patients.

Streptococcus pneumoniae has always been an important pathogen in the development of adult meningitis; now, however, this pathogen also is important in meningitis in children. In fact, the meningitis caused by *S. pneumoniae* is as common in children as meningitis caused by *Hemophilus influenzae* type B (HIB). The reason for this is the widespread use of HIB vaccine, which has led to a reduction of invasive HIB disease. In addition to the abovementioned risk factors, in young children daycare center attendance is a risk factor for the development of invasive pneumococcal disease.

The diagnosis of pneumococcal meningitis is made by obtaining CSF for Gram stain and culture. With all causes of bacterial meningitis, the CSF opening pressure and protein level generally are elevated, and the CSF glucose level is depressed. With pneumococcal meningitis, the CSF may have a greenish tint. A CSF leukocytosis is seen, with a predominance of polymorphonuclear (PMN) forms. In patients who have not received prior antimicrobials, the Gram stain reveals PMNs and gram-positive diplococci in the majority of cases. Cultures are positive for *S. pneumoniae* (see figure) in approximately 90% of persons who have received no treatment, but if prior antibiotics have been given, cultures are positive in less than half of patients. Latex agglutination tests for *S. pneumoniae* may be used when the Gram stain is negative; however, a negative latex agglutination test does not rule out bacterial meningitis.

Pneumococcal meningitis caused by susceptible strains can be treated with high-dose intravenous penicillin G. Alternatively, the physician should consider a third-generation cephalosporin, such as cefotaxime or ceftriaxone, since the incidence of β-lactam–resistant strains of pneumococci is increasing. Vancomycin should be added to the regimen initially if high-level β-lactam resistance is suspected. Vancomycin only variably penetrates the blood brain barrier: it should be used only in cases of high-level β-lactam resistance, or when there is no alternative therapy. Chloramphenicol recently has been shown to have a high failure rate in pneumococcal meningitis. Antimicrobials should be administered promptly in all suspected cases of bacterial meningitis.

The role of corticosteroid therapy in meningitis remains unclear. Studies have shown reduced neurologic sequelae in children with *H. influenzae* meningitis; however, although recent trials in children infected with *S. pneumoniae* demonstrated fewer neurologic sequelae, the difference was not statistically significant. In general, adjunctive corticosteroid therapy should be given to children with suspected bacterial meningitis.

The use of corticosteroids in adults remains controversial. Dexamethasone may be of benefit when organisms are visible on CSF Gram stain and there are signs of elevated intracranial pressure.

In the present patient, blood and CSF cultures grew *S. pneumoniae* after 24 hours of incubation. The organism was sensitive to penicillin. The patient was treated with intravenous ceftriaxone for 10 days; she did not receive any steroids. A CT scan of her sinuses was negative. The patient did well and ultimately was discharged from the hospital.

Clinical Pearls

1. Pneumococcal meningitis is associated with sinusitis, otitis media, skull fractures, and/or CSF leaks.

2. Pneumococcal endocarditis may result as a complication of pneumococcal meningitis.

3. The CSF in pneumococcal meningitis may have a greenish tint.

REFERENCES

1. Quagliarello VJ, Scheld WM: New perspectives on bacterial meningitis. Clin Infect Dis 1993; 17:603–610.
2. Townsend GC, Scheld WM: Clinically important trends in bacterial meningitis. Infect Dis Clin Pract 1995; 4:423–430.
3. Quagliarello VJ, Scheld VM: Treatment of bacterial meningitis. N Engl J Med 1997; 336:708–716.

PATIENT 9

A 20-year-old man with dysuria and scanty mucoid discharge

A 20-year-old man presents to his physician's office with a 5-day history of burning upon urination and a 3-day history of a clear urethral discharge. He denies fever, hematuria, and flank pain. He is sexually active with one female partner and does not use condoms. There is no history of prior sexually transmitted diseases. He takes no medications and has no medication allergies.

Physical Examination: Temperature 37.2°; pulse 72; respirations 12; blood pressure 110/72. General: healthy-appearing. HEENT: no abnormalities. Chest: clear bilaterally. Cardiac: no abnormalities. Abdomen: soft, nontender, no organomegaly. Extremities: no rashes, no deformities. Genitalia: normal; no testicular tenderness, masses, or genital lesions; mild meatal erythema with scanty mucoid discharge. Lymph nodes: no inguinal adenopathy.

Laboratory Findings: Urethral swab: 7 WBC/oil immersion field, no intracellular diplococci, negative gonorrhea culture, chlamydial antigen positive.

Question: What diagnosis could explain all the features of the patient's presentation?

Diagnosis: Nongonococcal urethritis

Discussion: As the name implies, nongonococcal urethritis (NGU) is an inflammation of the
urethra caused by conditions other than infection
with *Neisseria gonorrhoeae.* The majority of NGU
cases are infections caused by *Chlamydia trachomatis.* Other infectious etiologies of NGU include *Ureaplasma urealyticum, Trichomonas vaginalis,* and herpes simplex. In some cases, a cause is
never found. Other manifestations of *C. trachomatis* genital disease include epididymitis and proctitis in men; in women most chlamydial infections
are asymptomatic and, therefore, undiagnosed.
When the disease is symptomatic in females, it
most frequently presents as a mucopurulent cervicitis. Reiter's syndrome (which manifests as conjunctivitis), urethral cervicitis, arthritis, and muco-
cutaneous lesions can be seen in men and women
with chlamydial infection.

NGU presents with dysuria and a urethral discharge that tends to be scant and mucoid as opposed
to the copious, purulent secretions frequently encountered with gonorrhea. When the endourethral
exudate is Gram-stained and examined microscop-
ically, the presence of ≥ 5 PMN per oil immersion
field and the absence of *N. gonorrhoeae* are suggestive of NGU. Cultures for gonorrhea subsequently are negative. Definitive diagnosis of
chlamydial NGU can be made by demonstrating *C.
trachomatis* in culture or through detection of
chlamydial antigen in endourethral or endocervical
secretions. Screening tests for NGU include the
leukocyte esterase test, which is diagnostic when
positive, and an examination of the first 20 cc of the
first voided urine specimen in the morning, which
is suggestive of NGU when ≥ 10 PMN are present
per high-powered field. Physical examination is
generally nondiagnostic in NGU. Occasionally,
meatal erythema is seen, or the mucoid discharge
can be expressed by milking the urethra.

For uncomplicated urogenital infection with *C.
trachomatis,* a single 1-gram dose of azithromycin
can be used. This regimen assures maximal compliance. Alternative regimens include tetracycline

or doxycycline 100 mg PO bid for 7 days, or
ofloxacin 300 mg PO bid for 7 days. Erythromycin,
500 mg PO qid for 14 days is another option—this
regimen should be used for treatment in pregnancy.
Sexual partners of infected individuals should be
evaluated and treated, as well. Patients should be
reevaluated for other pathogens, such as *U. urealyticum* and *T. vaginalis,* if they do not respond to
initial therapy or if symptoms recur after treatment.

	Nongonococcal Urethritis	Gonococcal Urethritis
Symptoms	Asymptomatic, mild dysuria, frequent urination	Dysuria, frequent urination
Discharge	Mucoid	Purulent
Urethral Swab Gram Stain	≥ 10 PMN per high-powered field	PMN with gram-negative intracellular diplococci
Causative Agent	*Chlamydia trachomatis Ureaplasma urealyticum Trichomonas vaginalis* Herpes simplex (rarely)	*Neisseria gonorrhoeae*
Treatment	Azithromycin Doxycycline Erythromycin Ofloxacin	Cefixime Ceftriaxone Ciprofloxacin Ofloxacin

The present patient was treated with azithromycin,
on the basis of the positive chlamydial antigen on his
urethral specimen, prior to leaving the office. His sexual partner also was treated with azithromycin for an
asymptomatic *C. trachomatis* cervicitis.

Clinical Pearls

1. The most common cause of nongonoccocal urethritis is *Chlamydia trachomatis. Ureaplasma urealyticum, Trichomonas vaginalis,* and herpes simplex infections are seen with less frequency.

2. Reiter's syndrome can occur as a sequela to chlamydial nongonococcal urethritis.

3. Azithromycin 1 g, given as a one-time dose, is effective treatment for most cases of nongonococcal urethritis and assures patient compliance.

REFERENCES

1. Root TE, Edwards LD, Spengler PJ: Nongonococcal urethritis: A survey of clinical and laboratory features. Sex Trans Dis 1980; 7:59–65.
2. Martin DH, Mroczkowski TF, Dalu ZA, et al: A controlled trial of a single dose of azithromycin for the treatment of chlamydia urethritis and cervicitis. N Engl J Med 1992; 327:921–922.
3. Falagas ME, Gorbach SL: prostatitis, epididymitis, urethritis—IDCP Guidelines, Infect Dis Clin Pract 1995; 4:325–333.

PATIENT 10

A 40-year-old man with seizures

A 40-year-old Hispanic man is brought to the emergency department by ambulance after having a grand mal seizure at home. There is no history of recent illness, fever, headache, seizures, or head trauma. He drinks alcohol only occasionally and denies any other drug use. The patient has lived in the United States for 15 years, but occasionally has traveled to his previous home in Central America.

Physical Examination: Temperature 37.6°; pulse 88; respirations 12; blood pressure 132/76. General: somewhat somnolent, but appears comfortable. HEENT: no abnormalities. Chest: clear bilaterally. Cardiac: normal S_1S_2, no murmurs. Abdomen: soft, nontender, no masses. Extremities: no edema, no skin rashes. Neurologic: patient arousable; oriented to person, place, time; no cranial nerve abnormalities; no focal sensory or motor deficits.

Laboratory Findings: WBC 12,200/μl with 82% neutrophils, 15% bands, 2% monocytes, 1% eosinophils. Serum chemistries: normal. Urine analysis: 1^+ protein, no cells. CT scan of the head: multiple punctate calcifications; two enhancing cystic lesions with surrounding edema (see figure).

Question: What condition is suggested by the patient's clinical presentation?

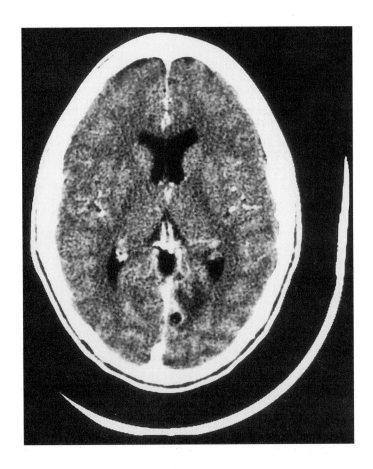

Diagnosis: Neurocysticercosis

Discussion: Cysticercosis is a tissue infection caused by the larval cysts of the cestode *Taenia solium*; when the central nervous system (CNS) is involved, the condition is termed neurocysticercosis. It is the most common parasitic infection of the CNS. The usual source of infection is the ingestion of undercooked pork. Although *T. solium* is found worldwide, infection with the organism is most frequently encountered in individuals from Mexico, South Central America, the Phillipines, and Southeast Asia. Person-to-person spread has been documented. Symptomatic *T. solium* disease is unusual unless the heart or central nervous system is involved.

In neuocysticercosis, the cysts act as space-occupying lesions and can cause hydrocephalus and/or seizures. The cysts, especially after many years, can degenerate, thereby evoking an inflammatory response that can result in seizures, cerebritis, or meningitis. The clinical presentation of neurocysticercosis is variable depending on the number of cysts and their size, location, age, and amount of associated inflammation. Signs of increased intracranial pressure such as headache, nausea, vomiting, or visual changes may be present. Cranial nerve abnormalities or focal neurologic findings also may be found. **Seizures,** which are the most common initial presentation of patients with neurocysticercosis, may be focal or generalized. Psychiatric disorders and changes in mental status are additional presenting signs of neurologic involvement. If the spinal cord is involved, symptoms of radiculopathy or cord compression may be seen. Since multiple cysts are common, patients can present with any combination of symptoms.

The diagnosis of neurocysticercosis is made using the clinical presentation and appropriate travel or exposure history in combination with CT or MRI findings. The CT scan generally shows multiple enhancing and nonenhancing cysts and, since some lesions are calcified, multiple punctate calcifications. These findings typically are observed at the grey/white matter juncture. MRI findings are similar, with multiple ring-enhancing cystic structures seen on T_1-weighted images. Lumbar puncture frequently reveals pleiocytosis, often with a lymphocytic predominance, of the cerebrospinal fluid. Eosinophils also may be observed. Cerebrospinal fluid protein generally is elevated, and the glucose is depressed. Serologic diagnosis has improved in the past few years with the development of immunoblotting techniques; however, these tests are less sensitive in patients with few or highly calcified cysts.

Medical therapy usually is the treatment of choice for neurocysticercosis. The most effective drugs are **praziquantel** or **albendazole** administered at high dosages. There often is a transient increase in symptoms during therapy due to cell death and increased inflammation. Dexamethasone may be administered during therapy to decrease these effects. Seizures should be controlled before, during, and after therapy with anticonvulsants, although the duration of therapy is the subject of debate.

The present patient was considered to have neurocysticercosis on the basis of the epidemiologic and radiographic findings. He was started on phenytoin and oral praziquantel. Since the patient did not have a heavy burden of cysts, dexamethasone was not given, as it can lower the praziquantel levels. The patient completed a 7-week course of therapy. Unfortunately, he was lost to follow-up, so his long-term response to therapy remains unknown.

Clinical Pearls

1. Neurocysticercosis is caused by central nervous system invasion by larval cysts of the cestode *Taenia solium*.

2. Neurological manifestations differ depending upon the size, number, and location of the cysts.

3. Praziquantel and albendazole are the drugs of choice in the treatment of neurocysticercosis.

REFERENCES
1. Del Brutto OH, Sotel J: Neurocysticercosis: An update. Rev Infect Dis 1988; 10:1075–1087.
2. Botero D, Tanowitz HB, Weiss LM, et al: Taeniasis and cysticercosis. Infect Dis Clin North Am 1993; 7:683–697.
3. Davis LE: Neurocysticercosis: Pathophysiology, diagnosis, and management. Infect Dis Clin Practice 1997; 6:358–365.

PATIENT 11

A 40-year-old alcoholic man with productive cough and right upper lobe opacities

A 40-year-old man presents to the emergency department with a 2-day history of fever to 39.4°C, shaking chills, and a cough productive of red sputum. The patient denies any previous medical problems, but admits to consuming 6–12 beers and smoking one pack of cigarettes per day.

Physical Examination: Temperature 39.6°; pulse 128; respirations 24; blood pressure 120/62. General: ill-appearing, poor hygiene. HEENT: minimal conjunctival and pharyngeal injection. Cardiac: normal S_1S_2, no murmurs. Chest: decreased breath sounds, dullness to percussion and egophony in right upper lobe. Abdomen: soft, nontender, no organomegaly. Extremities: no cyanosis, edema, or skin rashes.

Laboratory Findings: WBC 26,200/µl with 65% neutrophils, 25% bands, 8% lymphocytes, 1% monocytes. Sputum Gram stain: abundant polymorphonuclear leukocytes and short, gram-negative rods surrounded by a clear zone (see figure). Chest radiograph: right upper lobe opacity with bulging of the horizontal fissure.

Question: What diagnosis should be considered?

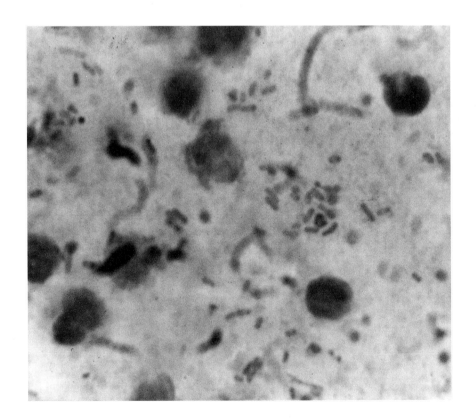

Diagnosis: *Klebsiella pneumoniae* pneumonia

Discussion: *Klebsiella pneumoniae* is an encapsulated, nonmotile, gram-negative rod that is a major cause of nosocomial infections. The organism also is a cause of community-acquired lobar pneumonias, most commonly seen in alcoholism, diabetes, and other forms of immunosuppression, and in chronic obstructive pulmonary disease.

Clinically, bronchopneumonia caused by *K. pneumoniae* presents similarly to the other community-acquired pneumonias, with an abrupt onset of fever, chills, cough, and hypoxemia. Rarely, infection is indolent, with a presentation similar to tuberculosis. Since the organism destroys lung tissue, the sputum may be bloody; classically, it has been described as **"currant jelly."** The sputum Gram stain often reveals an abundant number of polymorphonuclear leukocytes and short, gram-negative rods. These bacilli frequently are surrounded by an area of clearing, which is due to the presence of a mucoid capsule.

Since *K. pneumoniae* usually causes severe disease and rapidly develops resistance to antimicrobial agents, initial therapy typically consists of two agents, such as a third-generation cephalosporin plus a quinolone or aminoglycoside. The antipseudomonal penicillins are active against *Klebsiella* as well, and both meropenem and imipenem have been used successfully.

A complication of *K. pneumoniae* pneumonia is the development of **pulmonary gangrene**. Pulmonary gangrene is devitalization of a large amount of lung tissue, such as a segment or lobe, by necrosis and large vessel thrombosis. Patients with pulmonary gangrene require surgical debridement and/or drainage in addition to antimicrobial therapy.

The present patient was started on ceftazidime and ciprofloxacin for a severe, community-acquired pneumonia that appeared to be due to *K. pneumoniae* by Gram stain indices. The patient received intravenous antibiotics for 5 days and then left the hospital against medical advice.

Clinical Pearls

1. *K. pneumoniae* pneumonia generally occurs in persons with a history of alcoholism, diabetes mellitus, or chronic obstructive pulmonary disease.

2. The sputum often has a "currant jelly" appearance, and microscopic views typically reveal short, gram-negative rods surrounded by a zone of clearing.

3. Chest radiographs may show a bowed or bulging fissure in conjunction with a lobar opacity.

REFERENCES
1. Carpenter JL: *Klebsiella* pulmonary infections: Occurrence at one medical center and review. Rev Infect Dis 1992; 12:672–682.
2. Pugliese A, Domenico P, Cunha BA: *Klebsiella* infections. Infect Dis Practice 1993; 17:7–9.
3. Marrie TJ: Community-acquired pneumonia. Clin Infect Dis 1994; 18:501–515.

PATIENT 12

A 50-year-old man with fever, malaise, and inguinal adenopathy

A 50-year-old man presents with a 1-week history of fever, malaise, and tender, swollen inguinal lymph nodes on the left. He denies any other localized symptoms. He also denies trauma to the left leg. The patient is taking atenolol once daily for hypertension, and he is allergic to penicillin. He recently returned from a 2-month trip to Southeast Asia, but experienced no illness while traveling.

Physical Examination: Temperature 38.4°; pulse 68; respirations 10; blood pressure 130/80. General: uncomfortable-appearing. Cardiac: normal, regular rhythm, no murmur. Chest: clear. Abdomen: soft, nontender, no masses. Extremities: no edema, distal pulses intact. Genitalia: no penile lesions or discharge, no scrotal edema, no testicular tenderness or masses. Lymph nodes: inguinal matted and tender on left, with overlying erythema (see figure); no other lymphadenopathy. Skin: no rashes, no lesions.

Question: What is the likely diagnosis?

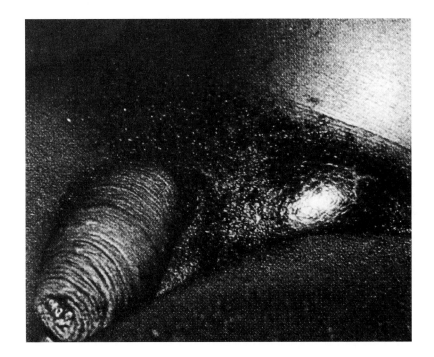

Diagnos

Discussi   granulomatous masses. A complication
(LGV) is :   lymphadenopathy or scarring is the de-
the L₁, L₂,   of genital elephantiasis. Another se-
tis. It is en   GV is the development of genital fistulas
Asia, Indi   es. In women and homosexual men, a
close sexu   of hemorrhagic proctocolitis can occur in
entry throu   er vaginal, or cervical infections. When
sure a sm   lvic nodes are involved, patients present
forms on t   back pain or abdominal pain that may
ticed, and   endicitis.
Systemi   is is made by clinical appearance and by
cur within   f *C. trachomatis* from bubo pus or other
Systemic   ssues; however, the organism is isolated
malaise, r   ut 30% of cases. Serologic testing, which
goenceph   d diagnostically, is not type-specific for
the lymph   ns of *C. trachomatis*, but titers are much
is depend   n those encountered with chlamydial non-
Since the p   l urethritis.
vulva, or a   nt of LGV is with oral **doxycycline,** 100
affected m   a day for 21 days. Alternatives include
discrete, t   cin and sulfisoxazole. Bubos should be
progress to   o prevent the formation of sinus tracts.
Eventually,   sent patient demonstrated the character-
"sign of the   arance of LGV, which was confirmed
both sides   lly. He was treated with a 3-week course
suggestive   xycycline. The patient's symptoms re-
Spontane   t his inguinal lymph nodes on the af-
months, but   were still palpable several months later.

Clinical Pearls

1. The primary lesion of lymphogranuloma venereum, a painless papule or vesicle at the site of innoculation, may go unnoticed.

2. The lymphadenopathy of LGV is unilateral in the majority of cases, as opposed to the typically bilateral adenopathy of herpes and syphilis.

3. Serologic testing is not specific for LGV strains of *C. trachomatis,* but titers are higher than those seen in chlamydial nongonococcal urethritis.

REFERENCES

1. Heaton ND, Yates Bell A: Thirty-year followup of lymphogranuloma venereum. Br J Urol 1992; 70:693–694.
2. Centers for Disease Control and Prevention: Recommendations for the prevention and management of *C. trachomatis* infections. MMWR 1993; 42:1–39.
3. Martin DH, Mroczkowski TF: Dermatologic manifestations of sexually transmitted diseases other than HIV. Infect Dis Clin North Am 1994; 8:537–582.
4. Fred HL: Case in point: Lymphogranuloma venereum. Hosp Prac (Off Ed) 1995; 30:31.

PATIENT 13

A 35-year-old alcoholic man with foul-smelling sputum

A 35-year-old man with a known history of alcohol abuse presents to the emergency department with a 3-week history of worsening, productive cough and fevers. The patient says he has had profuse sweating and believes he may be losing weight. The nursing staff notes that the patient is expectorating copious amounts of foul-smelling sputum. The patient had been hospitalized 1 year ago for pneumonia. His past surgical history is significant only for an appendectomy in childhood. The patient admits to drinking at least six alcoholic beverages and smoking one pack of cigarettes per day.

Physical Examination: Temperature 38.7°; pulse 110; respirations 22; blood pressure 120/62. General: unkempt, chronically ill-appearing. HEENT: poor dentition, mild pharyngeal injection. Chest: decreased breath sounds right middle and upper lobe, positive egophony. Cardiac: regular S_1S_2, soft systolic ejection murmur. Abdomen: soft, nontender; no organomegaly. Extremities: no edema; positive tinea pedis. Skin: multiple ecchymoses on the upper and lower extremities.

Laboratory Findings: Hct 31.2%; WBC 18,300/μl with 88% neutrophils, 9% bands, 3% monocytes; hemoglobin 10.4 g/dl. Sputum Gram stain: abundant WBC, abundant gram-positive cocci in chains, moderate gram-negative rods. Chest radiograph: right upper and middle lobe opacities plus cavitary lesion with air-fluid level in the right middle lobe (see figure).

Questions: What diagnosis should be considered? How should the patient be treated if the suspected diagnosis is confirmed?

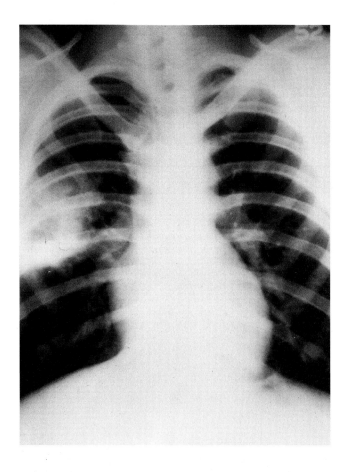

Diagnosis: Aspiration pneumonia with lung abscess

Discussion: A lung abscess can be primary, due to the aspiration of oropharyngeal contents, or secondary, as a result of another process such as subacute bacterial endocarditis, bacteremia, or subphrenic infection. Most lung abscesses are due to the aspiration of **anaerobic bacteria** such as *Peptostreptococcus* species, *Bacteroides*, and *Fusobacteria*, although a significant number of abscesses represent mixed anaerobic/aerobic infections. Aerobes implicated in the development of lung abscesses include *Staphylococcus aureus*, *Streptococcus pyogenes*, *Hemophilus influenzae*, *Mycoplasma pneumoniae*, and *Legionella* species. The majority of these cases are found in debilitated, hospitalized patients. *Actinomyces* species, *Nocardia* species, and *Entamoeba histolytica* also are occasionally responsible for abscess formation.

Persons at risk for the development of lung abscess are those who have an **altered level of consciousness,** such as alcoholics, drug abusers, and persons in a postictal state, and therefore have impaired airway-protection mechanisms. Others who have **impaired swallowing and gag reflexes** (e.g., persons who have had a cerebrovascular accident) are at increased risk for aspiration. **Gingivitis** and **pyorrhea** also are associated with abscess formation.

In patients who develop aspiration pneumonia with subsequent lung abscess, symptoms generally are present for several weeks. Common complaints include fevers (usually in the 101–102°F range), chills, sweats, weight loss, and pleuritic chest pain. **Cough** is present and generally productive; the **sputum** is described as foul in about 50% of patients. Physical examination findings are similar to those of pneumonia (e.g., egophony and fremitus). Poor dentition also may be seen, and clubbing of the fingers may be observed in those with long-standing disease.

Radiographic findings initially show **opacities**; **cavitary lesions** develop within approximately 2 weeks. These cavities may contain an air fluid level. Dependent portions of the lung are most often affected. Pleural effusions should be drained, with cultures sent for anaerobic and aerobic organisms. Blood cultures should be performed; however, more often than not they are negative, especially when anaerobic bacteria are the responsible pathogens.

Antimicrobial therapy is the mainstay of treatment for lung abscess. Since some strains of anaerobes are resistant to penicillin, many authorities feel that clindamycin should be used. If penicillin is chosen, it should be given in combination with metro-nidazole. Other alternatives include ampicillin/sulbactam, amoxicillin/clavulanate, imipenem, cefoxitin, chloramphenicol, and ticarcillin/clavulanate. A clinical response—for example, defervescence—usually is seen within 1 week, although radiographic abnormalities can persist for weeks to months. If clinical response does not occur, the clinician should look for causes, such as empyema (which requires chest tube placement), bronchial obstruction, large cavities, or an inappropriate choice of antibiotics. Bronchoscopy or transthoracic biopsy also can be considered at this point, to look for unusual or resistant organisms. The length of antibiotic therapy typically is 2–4 months.

Based on the present patient's history, physical exam, and chest radiograph, a diagnosis of lung abscess was determined. The patient initially was treated with 2 weeks of ampicillin/sulbactam with resolution of the fever and nightsweats. He was discharged with a prescription for amoxicillin/clavulanate which he was to continue for an additional 6 weeks. At his 1-month visit the patient felt well, and the abscess appeared smaller on chest radiograph.

Clinical Pearls

1. The clinical course of lung abscess frequently is indolent and, like tuberculosis, can present with fever, cough, weight loss, and night sweats.

2. Anaerobic bacteria are responsible for most lung abscess development.

3. Penicillin is no longer used alone in the empiric therapy of lung abscess in patients with moderate-to-severe illness because many of the anaerobes responsible for abscess development are resistant.

REFERENCES

1. Bartlett JG, Gorbach SL, Tally FP, Finegold SM: Bacteriology and treatment of primary lung abscess. Am Rev Respir Dis 1974; 109:510–584.
2. Bartlett JG: Anaerobic bacterial infections of the lung. Chest 1987; 91:901–907.
3. Hill MK, Sanders CV: Anaerobic disease of the lung. Infect Dis Clin North Am 1991; 5:453–466.

PATIENT 14

A 40-year-old diabetic man with necrotic cellulitis of the thigh

A 40-year-old man with a history of poorly controlled type II diabetes mellitus presents to the emergency department with a 3-day history of a skin infection on the anterior thigh. He denies trauma to the area, but it is the site of his insulin injections. The area was initially red and tender, but now blisters are developing. He has had fever as high as 40°C accompanied by shaking chills. His medications are neutral protamine Hagedorn insulin and enalapril; cephalexin was begun on day 3. He has no known drug allergies.

Physical Examination: Temperature 39.8°; pulse 132; respirations 20; blood pressure 98/72. General: ill-appearing. HEENT: no abnormalities. Cardiac: tachycardiac S_1S_2, no murmurs. Chest: clear. Abdomen: obese, soft, nontender, no organomegaly. Extremities: right thigh edematous, tense, and erythematous with multiple bullae; 3×3 cm necrotic area on anterior thigh. Lymph nodes: no regional lymphadenopathy.

Laboratory Findings: WBC 6200/µl with 50% neutrophils, 42% bands, 7% lymphocytes, 1% monocytes. Creatinine 2.0 mg/dl. Wound exudate: foul-smelling. Wound Gram stain: abundant WBC, gram-positive cocci, gram-positive bacilli, gram-negative rods.

Question: What is the likely diagnosis given this patient's presentation?

Diagnosis: Necrotizing fasciitis

Discussion: Necrotizing fasciitis is a life-threatening infection of the skin, subcutaneous tissues, and fascia. It can arise de novo, or develop after injury to the skin by trauma or surgery. Necrotizing fasciitis also can occur in association with intra-abdominal processes. Many patients have comorbid conditions, such as diabetes mellitus, peripheral vascular disease, corticosteroid therapy, or intravenous drug addiction.

Infections can be divided into two general types: fasciitis caused by group A hemolytic streptococci and sometimes staphylococci, and infections caused by mixed facultative and anaerobic organisms. Both types of infection present similarly, with rapidly progressive signs and symptoms of fever, chills, and **severely painful cellulitis** that may become bullous and/or gangrenous. Initially, the pain may be out of proportion to the severity of the cellulitis. In **streptococcal infection,** tissue gas is absent and a serous, odorless exudate is produced. In contrast, **mixed infections** due to anaerobes and Enterobacteriaceae produce a foul-smelling wound exudate and often generate gas in infected tissues. In both types of infection, tissue anesthesia may occur late in the clinical course secondary to thrombosis of blood vessels and nerve destruction. Surgical exploration of the affected area reveals extensive necrosis of the subcutaneous tissues and loss of the normal fascial planes.

Fournier's gangrene is a special case of necrotizing fasciitis involving the male or female genitalia. It is seen most often in older males, especially those with an underlying medical condition such as diabetes mellitus and a local predisposing factor such as a urinary tract infection or local soft-tissue infection. There is rapid progression of cellulitis involving the penis and/or scrotum, and in females, the vulva. The cellulitis may extend to the thighs and abdominal wall. Signs of systemic toxicity are present. Infection is caused by mixed organisms, including gram-negative rods such as *Escherichia coli* and *Pseudomonas aeruginosa,* facultative gram-positive cocci such as Enterococcus, and anaerobes like *Bacteroides* species and *Peptostreptococcus.*

The diagnosis of necrotizing fasciitis is made by history and clinical appearance, with a definitive diagnosis made at the time of surgical intervention. Gram-stained smears and cultures of wound exudate may help in selection of antimicrobial therapy.

Treatment of necrotizing fasciitis (including Fournier's gangrene) consists of prompt surgical debridement of the affected areas in combination with systemic antimicrobial therapy. Antibiotics chosen should be active against group A streptococci, facultative anaerobes, and anaerobic organisms. Possible regimens include ampicillin and gentamicin plus metronidazole (or clindamycin), ampicillin/sulbactam, or imipenem. Further surgical debridement often is required to remove necrotic tissue.

The present patient was suspected to have necrotizing fasciitis because of the appearance of the wound. A soft-tissue radiograph of the thigh demonstrated gas dissecting through tissue planes. Antibiotic therapy was initiated, and the patient was brought to the operating room where he underwent extensive debridement. The patient subsequently required several more debridements followed by skin grafting.

Clinical Pearls

1. Wound exudates in necrotizing fasciitis caused by group A streptococci are scant, serous, and odorless. In mixed infections gas is present, and exudate is foul-smelling.

2. Multiple surgical debridements in addition to antimicrobial therapy often are required for successful treatment of necrotizing fasciitis.

3. Fournier's gangrene, a necrotizing fasciitis of the genitalia, often is associated with an underlying condition such as diabetes mellitus or urologic infection.

REFERENCES
1. Loukhs SS: Fournier's gangrene. Surg Clin North Am 1994; 74:1339–1352.
2. Brook I, Frazier E: Clinical and microbiological features of necrotizing fasciitis. J Clin Microbiol 1995; 33:2382–2387.
3. Gorbach SL: Necrotizing skin and soft tissue infections. Part I: Necrotizing fasciitis. Infect Dis Clin Pract 1996; 5:406–411.

PATIENT 15

A 20-year-old man with right lower quadrant pain and
bloody diarrhea after travel to Mexico

A 20-year-old college student presents to his private physician's office with a 2-week history of crampy, right lower quadrant pain and bloody diarrhea. He has had low-grade fevers and complains of anorexia and weight loss of approximately 8 pounds. He denies nausea or vomiting. The patient recently returned from a Spring-break vacation in Mexico and admits to being careless about his food and water intake while away.

Physical Examination: Temperature 38°; pulse 90; respirations 14; blood pressure 112/76. General: healthy-appearing, no acute distress. HEENT: unremarkable. Cardiac: regular rate and rhythm; no murmurs. Chest: clear. Abdomen: soft; mild right lower quadrant tenderness; no guarding; no rebound; no organ enlargement; liver nontender. Extremities: no edema. Skin: no rashes.

Laboratory Findings: WBC: 10,800/µl with 78% neutrophils, 2% bands, 15% lymphocytes, 1% monocytes, 4% eosinophils. Liver function tests: normal. Stool for occult blood: positive. Direct examination of stool: see figure.

Question: What is causing the patient's symptoms?

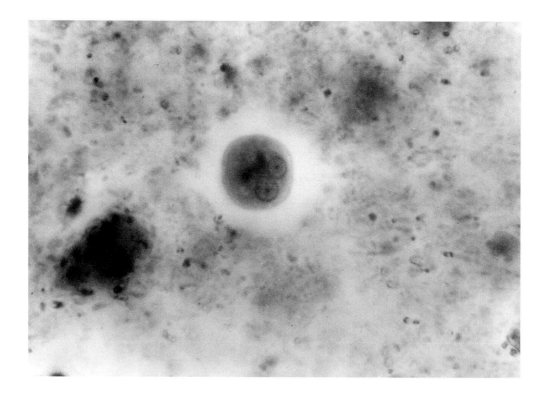

Diagnosis: Intestinal amebiasis

Discussion: Intestinal amebiasis is an illness caused by the free-living amoeba, *Entamoeba histolytica.* Since the cysts of the organism are transmitted via the **fecal-oral route**, infection with *E. histolytica* is endemic in developing nations that have poor sanitation. Natives and travelers to these areas experience a range of syndromes, from asymptomatic cyst passage to invasive colitis and/or liver abscess to rarely seen disseminated disease such as brain abscess or pericarditis.

When the cysts of *E. histolytica* are ingested, they are transported to the large bowel, where they excyst to the trophozoite form. These trophozoites cause ulceration of the intestinal wall, which causes the clinical symptoms. Depending on the number of organisms ingested, symptoms can range from mild abdominal pain with diarrhea (which is heme-positive), to a fulminant colitis with severe abdominal pain and bloody diarrhea. Fever is present in approximately 50% of patients.

An **amoeboma** is a localized, amebic infection that generally is found in the cecal area and can be mistaken for an acute appendix or a carcinoma. The organisms enter the portal venous system and invade the liver, where an amebic abscess may form. Symptoms of amebic liver abscess can be mild: low-grade fever, right upper quadrant pain, and weight loss are common. Leukocytosis and anemia frequently are present. Liver functions such as production of transaminase and alkaline phosphatase, are elevated, though the magnitude of the elevation often is low in comparison to the size of the abscess. *Amebic liver abscess can occur in the absence of intestinal symptoms and without evidence of the organism in the stool.*

The diagnosis of amebic colitis is made by examining stool specimens for the cysts or trophozoites of *E. histolytica.* Multiple stool specimens should be examined for the highest yield. If lower endoscopy is performed, scrapings and biopsy specimens should be obtained from the edge of an ulcer—where the organisms are more likely to be found. Serologic testing for antiamebic antibodies may be useful; titers are elevated in approximately 85% of persons with invasive disease. However, depending on the method used, it may be difficult to distinguish acute disease from past infection. CT scanning and abdominal ultrasonography are used to diagnose amebic liver abscess.

Therapy for invasive amebic colitis consists of metronidazole, which eliminates the trophozoite, followed by an agent active against cysts in the lumen of the bowel, such as diloxanide furoate, iodoquinol, or *paromomycin.* Amebic liver abscess can be treated with the same regimen. Alternatively, dehydroemetine with or without chloroquine has been used to eradicate the trophozoite phase. Most authorities advocate the treatment of asymptomatic cyst passers with a luminal agent alone.

Direct examination of the present patient's stool (see figure) revealed multiple cyst forms of *E. histolytica.* He was treated with a 10-day course of metronidazole, followed by diloxanide furoate. His symptoms resolved, and follow-up stool examinations were free of *E. histolytica.*

Clinical Pearls

1. Intestinal amebiasis can present as asymptomatic cyst passage, invasive colitis, or amoeboma. Liver abscess can be seen with or without evidence of intestinal infection.

2. When endoscopy is performed, scrapings and biopsies should be taken from the edge of an ulcer to maximize the chances of obtaining trophozoites.

3. Treatment of amebic colitis consists of both a tissue agent, such as metronidazole, and a luminal agent, such as diloxanide furoate, iodoquinol, or paromomycin.

REFERENCES
1. Drugs for parasitic infections. Medical Letter 1982; 24:5.
2. Reed SL, Wessel DW, Davis CE: *Entamoeba histolytica* infection in AIDS. Am J Med 1991; 90:269–270.
3. Ravdin JI: Amebiasis. Clin Infect Dis 1995; 20:1453–1466.

PATIENT 16

A 10-year-old boy with fever and obtundation

A 10-year-old boy is brought to the emergency department by his parents, who state they are unable to arouse him from sleep. The parents relate that the child has been sick with a viral illness for 2 days, with fever, headache, nausea, and vomiting. The child has a witnessed grand mal seizure in the emergency department.

Physical Examination: Temperature 39°; pulse 120; respirations 16. General: lethargic. HEENT: mild conjunctival injection, nuchal rigidity. Cardiac: regular rhythm, no murmurs. Chest: clear. Abdomen: soft, no masses, no organomegaly. Extremities: multiple insect bites and excoriations. Neurologic: drowsy but tremulous when stimulated; cranial nerves intact; deep tendon reflexes asymmetrical, plantar responses flexor.

Laboratory Findings: WBC 16,200/µl with 90% neutrophils, 1% bands, 8% lymphocytes, 1% monocytes. Cerebrospinal fluid (CSF): WBC 150/µl and RBC 1/µl with 92% neutrophils, 7% lymphocytes, 1% monocytes; protein 60 mg/dl; glucose 80 mg/dl. Gram stain: few WBC, no organisms seen.

Question: What diagnosis is most probable?

Diagnosis: Arboviral encephalitis

Discussion: Arboviruses (arthropod-borne viruses) are a group of enveloped RNA viruses responsible for a wide range of human disease. In the United States, arboviral encephalitis, which occurs both sporadically and epidemically, occurs mainly in four forms: St. Louis encephalitis, western and eastern equine encephalitis, and California encephalitis. The virus is transmitted to humans via the bite of **infected mosquitoes.** The spectrum of disease ranges from asymptomatic infection, to a mild viral syndrome, to an aseptic meningitis with encephalitis.

The four types of arboviral encephalitis share clinical manifestations, which also are similar to those of the more commonly encountered enteroviral aseptic meningitis. Signs and symptoms consist of **fever, headache, photophobia, nausea, and vomiting.** Myalgias and arthralgias typically are present. Lethargy and/or mental confusion are common. **Seizure activity** is most frequently observed in infants and young children, especially in those with California encephalitis.

Abnormalities on physical exam may include nuchal rigidity, muscular tremors, and focal neurologic findings such as cranial nerve abnormalities, paresis, and abnormal reflexes. **Conjunctival suffusion** is common and **skin rashes** similar to those seen in enteroviral infection also may be found.

Laboratory findings are nonspecific, consisting of a leukocytosis with a predominance of polymorphonucleotides; hyponatremia occasionally is seen secondary to inappropriate arginine dihydrolase secretion. The CSF is abnormal, with white cell counts in the hundreds (rarely, counts over $1000/\mu l$ are seen) and an early neutrophilic predominance; later, mononuclear cells present. Protein is mildly elevated, and the glucose is normal.

The diagnosis of arboviral encephalitis is made by demonstrating IgM antibody to the virus in the serum or CSF. Alternatively, rises in titers of acute and convalescent serum antibody may be shown. There is no specific therapy for arbovirus encephalitis, and treatment is entirely supportive. Mortality is low in California encephalitis; however, residual seizure activity is common. Mortality also is low in St. Louis and western equine encephalitis. Eastern equine encephalitis has a high mortality rate (about 50%), and children who survive this illness often are left with neurologic sequelae.

Arboviral encephalitis was suspected in the present patient on the basis of his symptoms and the known existence of mosquitoes in the area carrying the arbovirus. He was treated supportively. Ultimately, the diagnosis of California encephalitis was made using acute and convalescent antibody titers. After a long and complicated hospital stay, the patient was discharged home with a residual seizure disorder and multiple neurologic deficits.

Clinical Features of Arbovirus Encephalitis

Virus	Age Group	Signs/Symptoms	Laboratory Features
California encephalitis	Children <10	Seizures, focal neurologic signs, nausea/vomiting	Leukocytosis
Eastern equine encephalitis	Children Adults	Rapidly progressive encephalitis, brawny edema of face/extremities	Cloudy CSF, WBC $>1000/\mu l$, depressed CSF glucose
Western equine encephalitis	Infants Adults > 60	Tremors prominent, sequelae rare but severe	Normal WBC count
St. Louis encephalitis	Adults > 60	"Summer stroke" syndrome, dysuria (~20%), seizures, tremor	SIADH (~20%)

SIADH = syndrome of inappropriate secretion of antidiuretic hormone

Clinical Pearls

1. California encephalitis mainly affects children in the midwestern United States. Seizures are common both upon presentation and after resolution of the clinical illness.

2. Eastern equine encephalitis is localized to the eastern seaboard, where it strikes young children and adults. Mortality is high. A peculiar brawny edema of the face and extremities is a clinical clue.

3. St. Louis encephalitis is encountered in the East and Midwest, and patients present with neurologic symptoms and, often, dysuria.

4. Western equine encephalitis is found throughout the United States and affects infants and adults > 60 years old.

REFERENCES

1. Cunha BA: Acute encephalitis. Infect Dis Pract 1989; 12:1–11.
2. Tsai TF: Arboviral infections in the United States. Infect Dis Clin North Am 1991; 5:73–102.
3. Centers for Disease Control and Prevention: Arboviral disease—United States, 1994. MMWR 1995; 44:641–644.

PATIENT 17

A 35-year-old drug abuser with fever, lethargy, and left-sided weakness

A 35-year-old man with a known history of intravenous drug use is brought to the emergency department by a friend who states that the patient has been "sleepy" for a few days. The friend tells the nurse that the patient is HIV positive, but he is unable to give any other information. His past medical history, surgical history, and medications are unknown.

Physical Examination: Temperature 38.3°; pulse 84; respirations 14; blood pressure 100/68. General: thin; poor personal hygiene. HEENT: pupils reactive; questionable papilledema; oral thrush; mild pharyngeal infection. Neck: supple, cervical lymphadenopathy. Cardiac: regular rhythm, no murmurs. Chest: clear. Abdomen: soft, nontender, no organomegaly. Extremities: no clubbing, cyanosis, or edema. Neurologic: lethargic, but arousable; oriented to person and place; weakness of left upper and lower extremity.

Laboratory Findings: Hct 35.8%; WBC 6100/μl with 80% neutrophils, 18% lymphocytes, 2% monocytes; hemoglobin 12 g/dl. Electrolytes: normal. Chest radiograph: normal. Electrocardiogram: normal. Head computed tomography (CT) scan: multiple, enhancing, ring-shaped lesions associated with edema and moderate hydrocephalus (see figure).

Question: What diagnosis would explain the CT scan abnormalities?

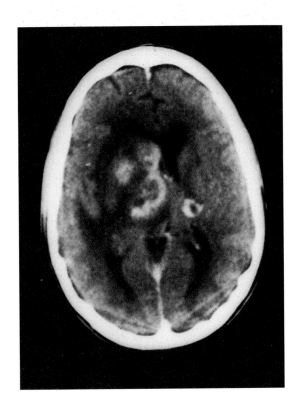

Diagnosis: Central nervous system toxoplasmosis

Discussion: Central nervous system (CNS) toxoplasmosis is caused by the obligate intracellular parasite *Toxoplasma gondii.* This organism is widespread in nature, and is found in many species of animals. Humans are infected when the oocysts from soil or the bradyzoites from undercooked meat are ingested. In the immunocompromised host, acute toxoplasmosis usually results in asymptomatic illness or lymphadenitis, though chorioretinitis, pneumonitis, myocarditis, and meningoencephalitis can occur. Infection is possible via intrauterine transmission, resulting in congenital toxoplasmosis.

CNS toxoplasmosis mainly occurs as a result of reactivation of *T. gondii* oocysts in a compromised host, such as a transplant recipient or an HIV-infected individual. It is the most common cause of cerebral mass lesions in patients with AIDS and is encountered most frequently in persons whose CD_4 count is less than $100/\mu l$. The variable clinical presentation of CNS toxoplasmosis includes fever, lethargy, mental status changes, headache, seizures, and focal neurologic deficits. Laboratory findings are nonspecific; analysis of cerebrospinal fluid frequently reveals only a pleocytosis, with protein at a mild-to-moderate elevation.

CT scans typically show **multiple, enhancing lesions** in the basal ganglia and corticomedullary regions, though any area of the CNS can be involved. The lesions usually are associated with cerebral edema, and there also may be a mass effect. Magnetic resonance imaging is more sensitive for smaller lesions, but neither study can differentiate toxoplasmosis from other CNS lesions such as lymphoma.

Definitive diagnosis of CNS toxoplasmosis is made by biopsy of brain lesions; however, this generally is not practical. In patients with AIDS who have a clinical presentation compatible with toxoplasmosis and serologic evidence of past exposure (IgG), **therapy is empiric.** Combination therapy with pyrimethamine and sulfadiazine, along with folinic acid to prevent bone marrow suppression, is used. Clindamycin and dapsone have been prescribed when sulfadiazine cannot be tolerated. Neurologic symptoms should stabilize or improve within 1 week of initiation of therapy; however, radiographic improvement may take several months. If there is deterioration, then a brain biopsy should be performed. Immunocompromised patients require lifelong suppression with pyrimethamine and sulfadiazine after initial treatment.

The present patient was begun empirically on clindamycin and sulfadiazine. His mental status improved over the subsequent 10 days. His CD_4 count was $20/\mu l$, and an HIV test was positive. A repeat CT scan done at the time of discharge on day 21 showed resolution of the cerebral edema and a decrease in the size of the lesions. Based on the patient's clinical and radiographic improvement on therapy, he was diagnosed with CNS toxoplasmosis and was continued on long-term suppressive therapy.

Clinical Pearls

1. Meat should be thoroughly cooked to avoid infection with *Toxoplasma gondii.*
2. Symptomatic CNS toxoplasmosis usually does not occur until the CD_4 count falls below $100/\mu l$.
3. Immunocompromised patients require life-long suppressive therapy.

REFERENCES
1. Cohn JA, McMeehing A, Cohen W, et al: Evaluation of the policy of empiric treatment of suspected Toxoplasma encephalitis in patients with the acquired immunodeficiency syndrome. Am J Med 1989; 86:521–832.
2. Porter SB, Sande MA: Toxoplasmosis of the central nervous system in the acquired immunodeficiency syndrome. N Engl J Med 1992; 327:1643–1648.
3. Richards FO, Kovacs JA, Luft BT: Preventing toxoplasmic encephalitis in persons infected with human immunodeficiency virus. Clin Infect Dis 1995; 21(Suppl 1):S49–56.

PATIENT 18

A 20-year-old homosexual man with a urticarial eruption and elevated liver function tests

A 20-year-old homosexual man presents to his physician's office with a 3-day history of headache, malaise, anorexia, nausea, and vomiting. He has had low-grade fevers in the 37.2°–38.3° range. On the day of his visit, he developed a urticarial eruption and diffuse arthralgias.

Physical Examination: Temperature 38°; pulse 110; respirations 12; blood pressure 112/64. HEENT: sclera anicteric; mild pharyngeal erythema; small, mobile cervical lymph nodes at posterior. Cardiac: regular rhythm, no murmurs. Chest: clear. Abdomen: soft; mild tenderness to deep palpation of right upper quadrant; liver edge smooth, palpable just below right costal margin; no splenic enlargement. Extremities: no edema. Skin: urticarial rash on trunk, extremities; no petechiae or purpura.

Laboratory Findings: Hct 37%; WBC 6500/μl with 45% neutrophils, 2% bands, 45% lymphocytes, 8% atypical lymphocytes; hemoglobin 12.3 g/dl. Bilirubin 2.5 mg/dl; PT and PTT normal; alanine aminotransferase 1326 mg/dl; aspartate aminotransferase 1258 mg/dl. Alkaline phosphatase: normal. Hepatitis serology: HBsAg positive; anti-HAV IgM negative; anti-HBs negative; anti-HBc IgM positive; HBcAg positive.

Questions: What is the likely diagnosis? How would you pursue it?

Diagnosis: Acute hepatitis B infection

Discussion: Hepatitis B virus is a DNA virus that is transmitted via contact with infected blood and other body fluids. Persons at high risk for acquiring hepatitis B include healthcare workers, dentists, intravenous drug users, homosexual males, infants of infected mothers, and hemodialysis patients. In approximately 50% of patients diagnosed with acute hepatitis B, no identifiable risk factor is found.

The incubation period of hepatitis B is 2–3 months. An unknown proportion of persons have **asymptomatic** infection. Others experience **nonspecific** prodromal symptoms consisting of fever, anorexia, nausea, vomiting, arthralgias, and myalgias. A small percentage of these patients experience an immune complex–mediated, serum sickness–like reaction featuring a symmetrical polyarthritis and a maculopapular or urticarial rash. Prodromal symptoms may persist for several weeks, but most resolve before the development of frank jaundice; nausea, vomiting, and anorexia may continue. Icterus may persist for 1–2 months before completely resolving. Physical examination may be completely normal, or tender hepatomegaly, posterior cervical adenopathy, and/or splenomegaly may be found. Rash and/or joint inflammation is observed in patients with the serum sickness–like presentation.

Laboratory abnormalities include **elevated serum transaminases**—up to 100 times the normal values, though peak values are not seen until the appearance of clinical jaundice—and elevated **serum bilirubin.** Alkaline phosphatase generally is in the normal range or only slightly elevated, and prothrombin time usually is normal except in severe disease. A lymphocytosis with atypical lymphocytes is seen on a complete blood cell count.

The definitive diagnosis of hepatitis B is made serologically (see table). The initial marker is **the presence of HBsAg,** which is elevated during the prodromal phase. HBsAg disappears within a few months, except in the chronic hepatitis B carrier state. **HBeAg,** which represents active viral replication as well as anti-HB core IgM, is seen during the acute phase of illness.

Treatment of hepatitis B infection is supportive. A safe and effective immunization is available and should be given to all individuals at risk for contracting hepatitis B.

The present patient was diagnosed with hepatitis B infection on the basis of positive serology. His symptoms spontaneously resolved over a 1-month period. His partner was found to be a chronic carrier of hepatitis B virus.

Hepatitis B Serology

	Anti-HBs	HBsAg	Anti-HBc IgM	Anti-HBc IgG	HBeAg	HBeAb
Acute hepatitis B	−	+	+	+	+	−
Hepatitis B carrier	−	+	−	+	−	+
Post hepatitis B infection	+	−	−	+	−	−
Hepatitis B vaccination	+	−	−	−	−	−

Clinical Pearls

1. Prodromal symptoms of hepatitis B are nonspecific, consisting of fever, malaise, anorexia, nausea, and vomiting. A few persons present with a serum sickness–like illness with a maculopapular or urticarial eruption and a symmetrical polyarthritis.

2. A lymphocytosis with atypical lymphocytes (usually between 5–20%) can be seen with acute hepatitis B.

3. Hepatitis B infection occasionally can cause a false positive heterophile antibody test.

4. Hepatitis B core antibody (IgG anti-HBc) is absent in persons immunized with the hepatitis B vaccine, but present in persons who have been infected with the virus.

REFERENCES
1. Wright TL, Lau JYN: Clinical aspects of hepatitis B virus infection. Lancet 1993; 342:1340–1344.
2. Hirschman SZ: Current therapeutic approaches to viral hepatitis. Clin Infect Dis 1995; 20:741–746.

PATIENT 19

A 30-year-old man with systemic toxicity and a progressive soft-tissue infection

A 30-year-old man presents to the emergency department with severe pain in the right calf. Three days earlier, he had required suturing of a deep laceration to his calf sustained in a motor vehicle accident. Initially he felt well, but over the past 48 hours he has had increasing pain and erythema of the lower leg and an intermittent, low-grade fever. He has not taken any medications.

Physical Examination: Temperature 37.8°; pulse 148; respirations 18; blood pressure 88/60. General: anxious, extremely diaphoretic. Head: unremarkable. Cardiac: tachycardic, regular rate and rhythm. Chest: clear bilaterally. Abdomen: soft, nontender, no masses, no organomegaly. Extremities: right calf edematous with deep erythema surrounding suture line; hemorrhagic bullae; brownish exudate from wound.

Laboratory Findings: Hct 37%; WBC 14,600/μl with 72% neutrophils, 22% bands, 6% lymphocytes. BUN 60 mg/dl; creatinine 2.8 mg/dl. Wound exudate Gram stain: few WBCs, abundant gram-positive rods. Right leg radiograph: gas in tissues.

Question: What is the likely cause of the gas in the tissues?

Diagnosis: Gas gangrene

Discussion: Gas gangrene is a rapidly progressive necrosis of muscle tissue. It also is known as clostridial myonecrosis because the majority of cases are caused by clostridial species. *C. perfringens* type A is the most common infecting organism; other *Clostridia* such as *C. septicum* and *C. novyi* also have been implicated. *C. perfringens* elaborates at least 12 toxins, and it is the alpha toxin that is responsible for the development of local and systemic illness.

C. perfringens and the other *Clostridia* species are ubiquitous. However, although many major and minor **traumatic wounds** are contaminated with these organisms, only a small number of wounds develop gas gangrene. In addition to traumatic injury, the **postoperative period**—especially in relation to gastrointestinal surgery—can be conducive to the development of this condition. It also can arise as uterine gas gangrene **postpartum** and after an **abortion**. Finally, gas gangrene can arise spontaneously.

The clinical manifestations of gas gangrene generally appear rapidly, usually within hours to a few days after the initial injury. The wound becomes severely painful. Edema of the wound often develops, and the site initially is pale and cooler than normal. A **thin, brownish exudate** with a sweetish odor may be present. Later, a deep erythema or bronzing of the skin may develop, along with hemorrhagic bullae. Systemic signs of infection include **tachycardia** with a minimally elevated temperature, hypotension, and renal failure. Despite these problems, patients remain remarkably alert, often with a feeling of impending doom. Tissue crepitance and the radiographic presence of tissue gas are not mandatory in the diagnosis of gas gangrene. Gram stain of the wound exudate reveals few polymorphonuclear leukocytes, but an abundance of **gram-positive rods.** Surgical exploration reveals that the muscle is noncontractile upon stimulation; it may appear pale externally, but internally it is beefy red. Later, it becomes frankly necrotic.

The diagnosis of gas gangrene is made on clinical grounds. Severe pain and edema in a wound are suggestive, especially when coupled with tachycardia in a patient who is afebrile. The watery, sweetish-smelling discharge with gram-positive rods is another clue. *C. perfringens* usually grows within 24 hours of culturing. *The presence or absence of tissue gas is an unreliable sign.* Definitive diagnosis is made at the time of surgery, and adequate surgical debridement is the mainstay of therapy. All necrotic muscle tissue must be removed. Adjunctive therapy includes antibiotics; a combination of penicillin and clindamycin is the treatment of choice. Since these wounds typically are contaminated by other bacteria, an aminoglycoside or third-generation cephalosporin should be added. Hyperbaric oxygen therapy remains controversial, and polyvalent antitoxin is no longer administered in most institutions.

The present patient was seen by an astute clinician who suspected a diagnosis of gas gangrene based on the clinical appearance of the wound and the Gram stain of the exudate. A radiograph of the site was performed, but there was no gas in the tissues. The patient was begun on antibiotics, and surgical debridement was performed. Although the patient lost a great deal of tissue from the area, he ultimately did well and was discharged.

Clinical Pearls

1. Gas gangrene should be suspected when pain in the wound is out of proportion to the physical findings or when there is unexplained tachycardia.

2. Exudate from the wound is watery and brownish, with a sweetish odor.

3. The presence or absence of gas in the tissues is not a reliable finding in gas gangrene.

4. Surgical debridement is the mainstay of therapy.

REFERENCES

1. Lehner PJ, Powell H: Gas gangrene. Brit Med J 1991; 303:240.
2. Lewis RT: Necrotizing soft tissue infections. Infect Dis Clin North Am 1992; 6:693–703.
3. Chapnick ER, Abter EI: Necrotizing soft tissue infections. Infect Dis Clin North Am 1996; 10:835–855.

PATIENT 20

A 40-year-old man with watery diarrhea after consumption of raw oysters

A 40-year-old man presents to his physician's office with a 2-day history of watery diarrhea. He denies blood or mucus in the stool, but states he has had severe abdominal cramps. His wife has begun to have similar symptoms. They were guests at a wedding several days ago, and although they ate different entrees, they both consumed shrimp, clams, and raw oysters during the cocktail hour. The patient had a tonsillectomy as a child, and has a history of hypertension. He is penicillin-allergic, and his usual medication is diltiazem.

Physical Examination: Temperature 38.3°; pulse 96; respirations 12; blood pressure 120/76. General: well-appearing, no acute distress. HEENT: dry oral mucosa. Chest: clear. Cardiac: regular rhythm, no murmurs. Abdomen: hyperactive bowel sounds; soft, minimal, diffuse tenderness upon deep palpation, but no guarding or rebound. Extremities: no cyanosis or edema. Skin: no rashes or lesions.

Laboratory Findings: Stool culture: oxidase-positive colonies. Thiosulfate-citrate-bile salts-sucrose (TCBS) agar culture: motile, curved, gram-negative rods (see figure).

Question: What condition should be considered as a cause of this patient's diarrhea?

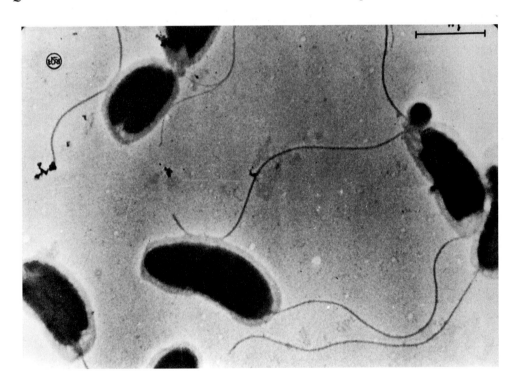

Diagnosis: Non-01 *Vibrio cholerae*

Discussion: The non-01 *Vibrio cholerae* are a group of organisms that are morphologically similar to, but biochemically different from, *V. cholerae* in that they do not agglutinate in 01 anti-serum. These strains of vibrios are found in warm, salt-water environments; in the United States they are found in the Gulf of Mexico. Disease in humans occurs when **infected raw or undercooked shellfish** are ingested.

Infection with non-01 strains of *V. cholerae* results in gastrointestinal disease, usually within 48 hours of ingestion. The most common clinical syndrome is that of **fever**; **copious, watery diarrhea**; and **abdominal cramps**. These symptoms are caused by the elaboration of cholera or cholera-like toxins. In addition, some *Vibrio* strains produce other factors which cause bloody or mucoid stools. Rarely, bacteremias, wound infections, and otitis media are seen.

Diagnosis is made by isolating the organisms from stool (or blood or wound exudate). A selective medium (TCBS) is required. A dietary history that includes raw shellfish ingestion should raise the suspicion of non-01 *V. cholerae* infection.

Illness usually is self-limited and lasts approximately 1 week. Therapy is supportive, with hydration and electrolyte replacement if necessary. Bacteremias, wound infection, and severe intestinal disease are treated with antimicrobials; experience in this area is limited, but the organism is sensitive *in vitro* to tetracycline, chloramphenicol, and quinolones.

The present patient was started empirically on ciprofloxacin by his physician for suspected food poisoning. By the time the organism was identified as a non-01 *Vibrio cholerae,* the patient was well and had returned to work. The patient's wife improved without any specific therapy.

Clinical Pearls

1. Non-01 *V. cholerae* gastrointestinal infection is caused by the ingestion of raw or undercooked shellfish that originated from warm, salt-water environments.

2. Selective media (TCBS) is required for the isolation of vibrios; however, stool cultures grown on nonselective media show a predominance of oxidase-positive colonies.

3. Illness is self-limited and usually does not require antimicrobials.

REFERENCES
1. Holmberg SD: Vibrios and aeromonas. Infect Dis Clin North Am 1988; 2:655–676.
2. Toxigenic non-01 group *Vibrio cholerae* infection acquired in Colorado. MMWR 1989; 38(2):1920–1924.

PATIENT 21

A 30-year-old man with tender inguinal adenopathy and painful penile ulcerations

A 30-year-old, sexually active man comes to your office complaining of painful penile ulcers and a tender groin. He denies fever, malaise, and anorexia and has no other systemic complaints. His past medical history is significant for syphilis, treated 2 years ago, and genital herpes infection.

Physical Examination: Temperature 37°; pulse 60; respirations 12; blood pressure 120/70. General: no distress. Mouth: normal. Cardiac: normal. Chest: clear. Abdomen: soft, nontender, no organomegaly. Lymph nodes: tender right inguinal adenopathy. Genitalia: three painful, ragged ulcerations 1 cm in diameter.

Laboratory Findings: Hct 36%; WBC 8000/μl with 60% polymorphonuclear cells, 40% lymphocytes; Veneral Disease Research Laboratory (VDRL) test: negative. Gram stain of exudate from ulcer: gram-negative coccobacilli (see figure below).

Question: What diagnosis should be considered?

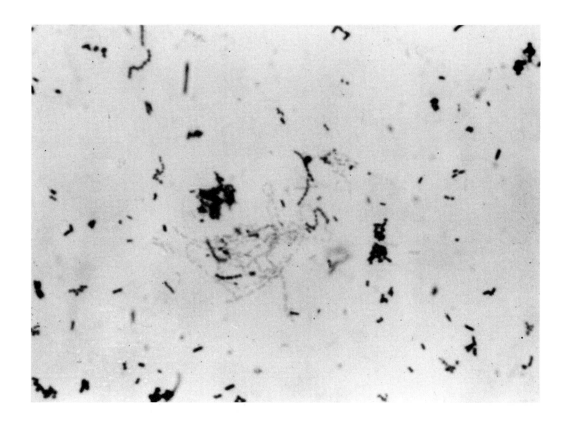

Diagnosis: Chancroid

Discussion: Chancroid is a sexually transmitted, ulcerative disease caused by *Haemophilus ducreyi*. The incubation period is about 7 days, but can vary from 2 days to several weeks. Initially, a small papule on an erythematous base may appear; it often is unnoticed by the patient until its rapid transformation into a painful ulcer with undermined, ragged edges and a friable base. Systemic symptoms are absent, but 50% of patients develop tender **unilateral inguinal adenopathy**. The number of ulcers varies: men tend to have single ulcers whereas women have multiple (10–15) lesions.

The diagnosis of chancroid is made by culturing the ulcer base. Gram stain of the ulcer exudate reveals gram-negative coccobacilli in a "school-of-fish" pattern. The patient also should be screened for syphilis by serology and darkfield examination of exudate, since simultaneous disease can occur. As many as 10% of patients with chancroid may be coinfected with syphilis or herpes simplex virus (HSV). Chancroid is the most common genital ulcer disease in Africa and Asia, but is seen less often in the United States and Europe. Contact with a prostitute is a risk factor for both chancroid and syphilis. Chancroid must be distinguished from other causes of genital ulcer adenopathy syndrome such as syphilis, HSV, lymphogranuloma venereum, and donovanosis. The presence of genital ulcer disease increases the chance of acquiring human immunodeficiency virus (HIV) infection through heterosexual intercourse.

The treatment of choice for chancroid is one dose of **ceftriaxone**, 250 mg. Alternative therapies are: a 7-day course of erythromycin or amoxicillin-clavulanic acid, a 3-day course of ciprofloxacin, or a single-dose treatment of 1 gm PO azithromycin.

All patients with chancroid should be tested for HIV, and if negative the test should be repeated in 3 months. Patients coinfected with HIV and chancroid may require longer treatment. The ideal regimen for HIV-positive individuals is not known. The 7-day erythromycin regimen has been successful in some patients, but a paucity of data is available on the use of ceftriaxone or azithromycin.

Once patients begin therapy, symptoms improve within 3 days. The ulcers heal slowly, but usually decrease in size within 7 days; large ulcers may require several weeks for complete healing. Tender inguinal adenopathy also resolves slowly over several weeks. Healing is slower in HIV-positive patients, and treatment failures have occurred. Sexual partners should be treated if they had sexual contact with the patient with chancroid during the 10 days before the appearance of lesions. Pregnant women should be treated with erythromycin. Chancroid does not appear to adversely affect pregnancy or fetus.

In the present patient, *H. ducreyi* was cultured from the ulcer, and Gram stain showed the typical gram-negative coccobacilli. HIV and VDRL tests were negative. Both the patient and his sexual partner were treated with ceftriaxone.

Clinical Pearls

1. Chancroid ulcers are painful, nonindurated lesions with ragged, undermined edges and a friable base.

2. Gram stain of the ulcer exudate reveals gram-negative coccobacilli in a characteristic "school-of-fish" pattern.

3. The presence of chancroid increases the chance of acquiring HIV infection through heterosexual intercourse.

REFERENCES
1. Jessamine PG, Ronald AR: Chancroid and the role of genital ulcer disease in the spread of human retrovirus. Med Clin North Am 1990; 74:1417–1431.
2. Schmid GP: Treatment of chancroid. Rev Infect Dis 1990; 12 (Suppl 6):580–589.
3. Engelkens HJH, Stolz E: Genital ulcer disease. Int J Dermatol 1993; 32:169–181.

PATIENT 22

A 25-year-old man with fever, a cold right foot, and a history of drug abuse

A 25-year-old man comes to the emergency department complaining of fever of 1-week duration accompanied by malaise, anorexia, and arthralgias. Yesterday he noted the onset of severe pain in his right foot. Past medical history is notable for an 8-year history of heroin abuse.

Physical Examination: Temperature 39°; pulse 110; respirations 20; blood pressure 120/80. General: ill-appearing. HEENT: unremarkable. Cardiac: S_1S_2 grade II/VI systolic murmur. Chest: clear. Abdomen: soft, nontender, positive bowel sounds, no organomegaly. Extremities: right foot cold and cyanotic, absent dorsalis pedis pulse.

Laboratory Findings: WBC 18,000/μl with 90% neutrophils, 5% bands, 5% lymphocytes; platelets 150,000/μl. Urinalysis: RBC 50/hpf, WBC 20/hpf, 2+ protein. Chest radiograph: no opacities. Blood cultures: two sets positive for yeast-like organisms (see figure).

Question: What is your diagnosis?

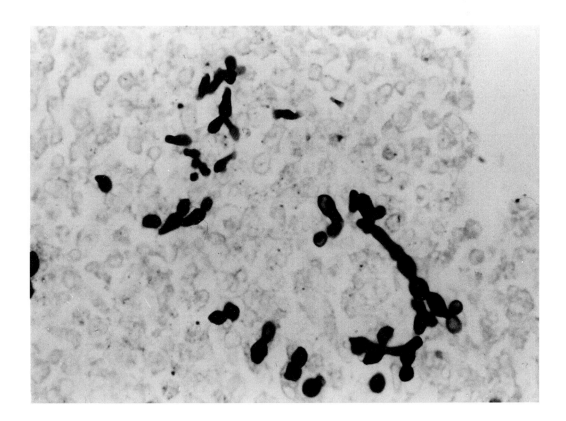

Diagnosis: *Candida* endocarditis

Discussion: Fungal endocarditis occurs in a variety of clinical settings, such as narcotic addiction, prolonged intravenous antimicrobial therapy, and immunosuppression, as well as after cardiac surgery. Fungal endocarditis accounts for 12–20% of cases of endocarditis in **intravenous drug users.** *Candida parapsilosis* accounts for more than half of these infections; *C. albicans* or *C. stellatoidea* for about 13%. Other less common fungal pathogens that have been reported to cause endocarditis in this setting are *C. krusei, C. tropicalis, C. guillermondii, Aspergillus* spp., *Torulopsis glabrata, Mucoraceae,* and *Saccharomyces.*

Candida endocarditis occurring after cardiovascular surgery is most often caused by *C. albicans,* non-*albicans Candida* spp., or *Aspergillus* spp. *C. albicans* is the most common fungal pathogen causing fungal endocarditis in patients receiving prolonged intravenous therapy. Fungal endocarditis in the immunosuppressed patient typically is due to *Aspergillus* spp.

The symptoms and physical findings of fungal endocarditis do not differ from bacterial endocarditis except for the occurrence of **large emboli** in the former. More than 75% of patients with *Candida* endocarditis have fever, heart murmur, and petechiae. Osler's nodes, Janeway lesions, splinter hemorrhages, and Roth's spots occur less frequently. Many patients have hepatosplenomegaly, hematuria, and proteinuria on presentation. Patients with fungal endocarditis usually have large vegetations, and peripheral embolization is the presenting manifestation in more than 40% of patients. Embolization of the brain, spleen, kidneys, and extremities are most common.

Routine laboratory data may reveal a leukocytosis or leukopenia, anemia, elevated liver function abnormalities, and hematuria and proteinuria in 50–75% of patients. Blood cultures are positive in up to 90% of cases of *C. albicans* or non-*albicans Candida* endocarditis, whereas blood cultures in *Aspergillus* endocarditis are positive in only 11%.

Candida endocarditis most commonly involves the **aortic and mitral valve.** The major complications are valve perforation, congestive heart failure, and major embolic events to the brain, kidney, extremities, and myocardium. The average size of fungus vegetations is reported to be about 2 cm—easily visualized by echocardiography.

The treatment of *Candida* endocarditis is **amphotericin B** combined with **valve replacement.** Amphotericin B should be administered for a minimum of 6 weeks and the patient closely followed for relapse. Ideally, early valve replacement—before the onset of embolic complications, heart failure, or ring abscess formation—should be performed.

The present patient had *C. parapsilosis* endocarditis. A transesophageal echocardiogram revealed a large vegetation on the aortic valve. Amphotericin B was begun, and the patient underwent aortic valve replacement.

Clinical Pearls

1. The most common organism causing fungal endocarditis in narcotic addicts is *Candida parapsilosis.*
2. Fungal endocarditis is an absolute indication for valve replacement.
3. A major complication of *Candida* endocarditis is the occurrence of large arterial emboli.

REFERENCES

1. Galgiani JN, Stevens DA: Fungal endocarditis: Need for guidelines in evaluating therapy. J Thorac Cardiovasc Surg 1977; 73:293–296.
2. Edwards JE, Jr: Invasive *Candida* infections. N Engl J Med 1991; 324:1060–1062.
3. Weems JJ Jr: *Candida parapsilosis:* Epidemiology, pathogenicity, clinical manifestations and antimicrobial susceptibility. Clin Infect Dis 1992; 14:756–766.

PATIENT 23

A 25-year-old diabetic woman with deteriorating mental status

A 25-year-old insulin-dependent diabetic is brought to the emergency department by her parents. She has been complaining of headache and facial pain for more than a week, and she noted some swelling over her left eye yesterday. This morning her parents found her obtunded, febrile, and with bilateral orbital swelling. Past medical history is notable for poorly controlled diabetes mellitus.

Physical Examination: Temperature 39.8°; pulse 130; respirations 30; blood pressure 120/80. General: lethargic, with bilateral orbital swelling. HEENT: bilateral proptosis and chemosis; black necrotic plaque in nasal turbinate. Neck: supple. Cardiac: regular rhythm, no murmur. Lungs: clear. Abdomen: soft, nontender, normal bowel sounds. Neurologic: cranial nerves II–XII intact.

Laboratory Findings: WBC 15,000/μl with 85% neutrophils, 5% bands, 10% lymphocytes. Glucose 500 mg/dl. Urinalysis: 4+ glucose, 4+ ketones.

Question: What diagnosis should be considered?

Diagnosis: Rhinocerebral mucormycosis

Discussion: Rhinocerebral mucormycosis is a life-threatening, invasive infection caused by the saprophytic fungi of the order *Mucorales* that occurs primarily in acidotic diabetics, neutropenic patients with leukemia, and transplant patients. Another recently recognized risk factor for mucormycosis is the administration of deferoxamine to patients on hemodialysis. The most common pathogenic genera causing rhinocerebral mucormycosis are *Rhizopus, Rhizomucor, Absidia, Mucor, Mortierella,* and *Cunninghamella*. These organisms are ubiquitous in the environment and are involved in the decay of organic material. The airborne spores are inhaled into the lungs or deposited into nasal turbinates where germination and proliferation occurs, followed by invasion of tissue. The fungus has a predilection for blood vessels, resulting in tissue necrosis and thrombosis that produce characteristic black, necrotic plaques.

In addition to rhinocerebral mucormycosis, these fungi may cause a number of other clinical entities such as pulmonary, gastrointestinal, central nervous system, cutaneous, and disseminated mucormycosis. Each form has different predisposing conditions. Disseminated disease occurs most often in severely immunocompromised patients, such as bone marrow transplant recipients or patients with acute leukemia.

Rhinocerebral mucormycosis is the most common form seen in diabetics. The infection begins in the nasal passages, extends into the paranasal sinuses, and spreads through the cribiform plate to the frontal lobes of the brain. Patients typically complain of headache, facial pain, and orbital swelling. Periorbital ecchymosis, chemosis, proptosis, and eye discharge frequently are seen when there is retro-orbital involvement. Necrotic lesions on the palate and in nasal passages is seen in 40% of patients. Mental status changes and cranial nerve abnormalities may be noted. There can be loss of vision due to thrombosis of the retinal artery. Involvement of cranial nerves V and VII occurs with progression of disease. Other serious complications include cerebral abscess, cavernous sinus, and internal carotid artery thrombosis.

The diagnosis is suggested by computed tomography scan or magnetic resonance imaging of the sinuses and orbits. Laboratory tests are nonspecific. Biopsy of necrotic plaques reveals characteristic broad, nonseptate hyphae branching at right angles.

Pulmonary mucormycosis occurs in severely immunocompromised patients, usually with neutropenia secondary to chemotherapy for acute leukemia. Patients present with fever and dyspnea. Hemoptysis can occur from tissue necrosis and, rarely, fatal pulmonary hemorrhage develops. The chest radiograph is nonspecific, but often shows cavitating lesions. Diagnosis depends on demonstration of the characteristic hyphae in tissue.

Gastrointestinal mucormycosis is found in patients suffering from severe malnutrition. The most common sites of involvement are the stomach, ileum, and colon. The fungus probably enters the gastrointestinal tract via food. Patients develop severe abdominal pain, nausea, vomiting, fever, and hematochezia. Most cases rapidly are fatal.

Cutaneous mucormycosis was reported due to contaminated elastic bandages in the 1970s. Patients developed cellulitis underneath the bandage due to direct inoculation of fungi into the skin. Cutaneous mucormycosis also has occurred after intramusuclar injections and after trauma. Both epidermis and dermis are involved, and the skin shows a characteristic necrosis due to vascular thrombosis.

Central nervous system mucormycosis occurs rarely and only in severely debilitated patients. Fungus enters the brain via the nose or paranasal sinuses or as a result of head trauma. Patients present with decreasing consciousness and development of focal neurologic deficits. Diagnosis is made at biopsy. There is necrosis of the dura and brain.

The treatment of invasive mucormycosis is **amphotericin B** combined with aggressive **surgical debridement** of necrotic tissue. There are several reports of the successful use of liposomal amphotericin B to treatment mucormycosis. The oral azole agents—fluconazole and itraconazole—are ineffective against these fungi. Despite early treatment with amphotericin B, invasive mucormycosis has a high mortality rate.

In the present patient, biopsies of the black plaques revealed broad, nonseptate hyphae identified as a *Rhizopus* species (see figure next page). Treatment for rhinocerebral mucormycosis was initiated. However, despite surgical intervention and liposomal amphotericin B, the patient died.

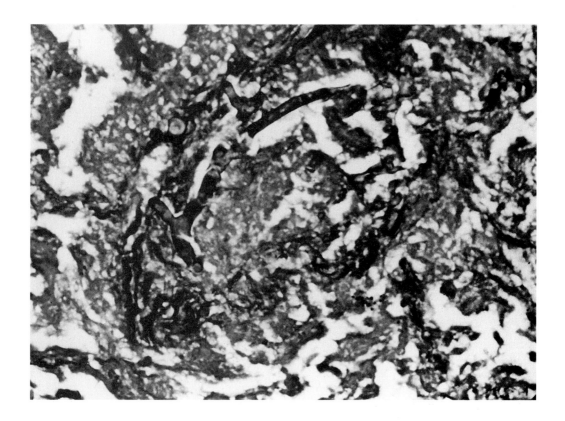

Clinical Pearls

1. *Rhizopus* and *Rhizomucor,* the primary fungi causing rhinocerebral mucormycosis, have broad, nonseptate hyphae branching at right angles. They are easily differentiated from *Aspergillus* hyphae, which are thin and septate and branch at acute angles.

2. A newly recognized risk factor for mucormycosis is dialysis patients receiving deferoxamine for chelation therapy.

3. None of the azole drugs are active against mucormycosis. Amphotericin B remains the only therapy.

REFERENCES

1. Blatt SP, Lucey DR, Deltoff D, et al: Rhinocerebral zygomycosis in a patient with AIDS. J Infect Dis 1991; 164:215–216.
2. Sugar AM: Mucormycosis. Clin Infect Dis 1992 (Suppl 1); S126–S129.
3. Tone-Cisneros J, Kusne S, Martin M, et al: Rhinocerebral mucormycosis after liver transplantation. Transplant Sci 1992; 2:63–64.
4. Ballaert JR, de Locht M, van Cutsem J, et al: Mucormycosis during deferoxamine therapy is a siderophore-medicated infection on vitro and in vitro animal studies. J Clin Invest 1993; 91:1976–1979.
5. Ericsson M, Annilco M, Gustafsson H, et al: A case of chronic progressive rhinocerebral mucormycosis treated with liposomal amphotericin B and surgery. Clin Infect Dis 1993; 16:585–586.

PATIENT 24

A 10-year-old boy with fever and rash

A 10-year-old boy is brought to your office because of a rash and fever of 2-day duration. The rash began on the face and spread to the neck, chest, and extremities; it was accompanied by fever to 38°C and malaise. The patient denies coryza, pruritus, swollen glands, and sore throat. Past medical history is unremarkable.

Physical Examination: Temperature 38°; pulse 90; respirations 14; blood pressure 100/60. General: well-appearing, no acute distress. HEENT: absence of pharyngitis and conjunctivitis. Neck: supple. Cardiac: regular rhythm, no murmur. Abdomen: soft, nontender, no organomegaly. Skin: diffuse, fine, maculopapular rash on face, neck, chest, and extremities.

Laboratory Findings: Hct 36%; WBC 6000/μl with 60% neutrophils, 40% lymphocytes; platelets 250,000/μl; hemoglobin 14 g/dl.

Question: What diagnosis should be considered?

Diagnosis: Echovirus exanthem

Discussion: Echoviruses along with coxsack-ievirus group A and B comprise the genus *Enterovirus*. The majority of infections caused by enteroviruses are asymptomatic or cause mild, nonspecific, febrile illnesses. However, a number of distinctive syndromes can occur (see table). Echoviruses cause a variety of **exanthems,** most commonly **maculopapular, rubelliform,** or **morbilliform** in nature. Epidemics of these exanthems can occur in children. Typically the rash begins simultaneously with the fever and appears first on the face before spreading downward to the neck, chest, and extremities. Echovirus exanthems can be distinguished from measles by the absence of coryza, Koplik spots, and conjunctivitis. Echovirus 16 causes Boston exanthem, a roseola-like illness characterized by fever with the appearance of a macular rash on defervescence. Petechial and purpuric rashes also have been seen with echovirus 9 and coxsackievirus A9 mimicking meningococcal disease.

Enterovirus is a common cause of aseptic meningitis, a syndrome characterized by meningeal irritation and cerebrospinal fluid (CSF) pleocytosis. Usually there is a preceeding prodromal illness followed by the onset of severe headache, meningismus, fever, and pharyngitis. About one third of patients have positive Kernig and Brudzinski signs. The peripheral WBC usually is normal or depressed. The CSF generally is clear, with 10–500 cells/μl—predominantly lymphocytes, although early on there may be a predominance of polymorphonuclear leukocytes. The CSF glucose is normal, and the CSF protein is mildly elevated.

A variety of other clinical syndromes can be caused by enteroviruses, including acute respiratory illnesses, encephalitis, herpangina, epidemic pleurodynia, myopericarditis, and acute hemorrhagic conjunctivitis.

The present patient had self-limited, febrile illness and maculopapular rash caused by echovirus. The diagnosis was made by demonstrating a fourfold rise in echovirus antibody convalescent titers obtained 3 weeks after the onset of the illness. He slowly improved over the next few days, and the fever and rash resolved 7 days after the onset of infection.

Syndrome	Enterovirus
Aseptic meningitis	Echovirus, coxsackievirus A & B
Encephalitis	Echovirus, coxsackievirus A & B
Paralysis	Echovirus, coxsackievirus A & B
Exanthem	Echovirus, coxsackievirus A & B
Herpangina	Coxsackievirus group A
Hand-foot-mouth disease	Coxsackievirus group A
Epidemic conjunctivitis	Coxsackievirus group A
Pleurodynia	Coxsackievirus group B
Myocarditis/pericarditis	Coxsackievirus group B
Chronic meningoencephalitis in agammaglobulinemics	Echovirus

Clinical Pearls

1. Enteroviral rashes may mimic rubella, measles, or meningococcal disease.

2. Herpangina, which is caused most commonly by coxsackievirus group A but also by group B1–5 and echoviruses, is a painful vesicular exanthem of the soft palate often accompanied by fever.

3. Coxsackievirus A16 causes hand-foot-mouth disease characterized by painful vesicles in the oral cavity and on the hands and feet accompanied by fever.

REFERENCES
1. Hall CB, Cherry JD, Hatch MH, et al: The return of Boston exanthem: Echovirus 16 infections in 1974. Am J Dis Child 1977; 131:323.
2. Jin O, Sole MJ, Butany JW, et al: Detection of enterovirus RNA in myocardial biopsies from patients with myocarditis and cardiomyopathy using gene amplification by polymerase chain reaction. Circulation 1990; 82:8–16.
3. Berlin LE, Rorabaugh ML, Heldrich F, et al: Aseptic meningitis in infants less than two years of age: Diagnosis and etiology. J Infect Dis 1993; 168:888–892.

PATIENT 25

A 10-year-old boy with a painful, swollen foot

A 10-year-old boy comes to the emergency department complaining of pain and swelling of 10-day duration in his right foot. About two weeks ago he sustained a puncture wound to this foot while wearing sneakers. Two days later he noted pain and swelling and was treated with cephalexin by his pediatrician. However, his symptoms persisted, and he is now unable to walk on the foot. The patient denies fever, chills, or malaise. Past medical history is unremarkable. He has no known allergies.

Physical Examination: Temperature 37°; pulse 90; respirations 12; blood pressure 110/60. General: no acute distress. HEENT: no abnormalities. Cardiac: regular rhythm, no murmur. Chest: clear. Abdomen: soft, nontender, positive bowel sounds. Extremities: plantar surface of right foot erythematous, tender, and swollen.

Laboratory Examination: Hct 36%; WBC 18,000/μl with 90% neutrophils, 5% bands, 5% lymphocytes; platelets 200,000/μl; ESR 70 mm/hr. Radiograph of foot: negative. Technetium bone scan: positive.

Question: What is your diagnosis?

Diagnosis: *Pseudomonas* osteochondritis

Discussion: *Pseudomonas aeruginosa* is the most common cause of osteochondritis involving the cartilage, small joints, and bones of the foot. *Pseudomonas* osteochondritis was first described after puncture wounds of the foot in children wearing sneakers, and *Pseudomonas* has been isolated from the soles of the sneakers. Patients usually present a week after the injury, and therapy with routine antibiotics used for cellulitis often has failed. There may be early improvement in pain and swelling after the puncture wound, followed by worsening symptoms several days later. The most common presentation is a swollen, tender foot. Examination of the plantar surface may reveal cellulitis and sometimes drainage. Patients usually are afebrile, and systemic symptoms typically are absent. Radiographs may be negative early on in the disease, but **bone scans** should be positive. The diagnosis is confirmed by growing *P. aeruginosa* from an aspiration of the affected area. Infection can involve the proximal phalanges/metatarsals, tarsal bones, and calcaneus.

Treatment consists of **surgical debridement** and **antipseudomonal antibiotics,** such as pipericillin or ceftazidime, combined with gentamicin. The length of therapy is controversial. Some patients respond to a short course (1–2 weeks); however, relapses can occur.

In the present patient, the radiograph of the foot was negative for osteomyelitis, but a bone scan was positive. Aspiration of the foot revealed a small amount of purulent material which grew *P. aeruginosa*. He was treated with a 3-week course of pipericillin and gentamicin plus surgical debridement, with a good response.

Clinical Pearls

1. Sneakers are the source of *Pseudomonas aeruginosa* in osteochondritis following puncture wounds.

2. Systemic symptoms such as fever and chills usually are absent.

3. Technetium scan almost always is positive in *Pseudomonas* osteochondritis, but radiographs can be negative.

REFERENCES

1. Jacobs RF, Adelman L, Sack CM, et al: Management of *Pseudomonas* osteochondritis complicating puncture wounds of the foot. Pediatrics 1982; 69:432–435.
2. Fisher MC, Goldsmith JF, Gilligan PH: Sneakers as a source of *Pseudomonas aeruginosa* in children with osteomyelitis following puncture wounds. J Pediatr 1985; 106:607–609.
3. Jacobs RF, McCarthy RE, Elsen JM: *Pseudomonas* osteochondritis complicating puncture wounds of the foot in children: A 10 year evaluation. J Infect Dis 1989; 160:657–661.

PATIENT 26

A 15-year-old boy bitten by a dog

A 15-year-old boy comes to the emergency department with pain and redness that developed in the injured arm 18 hours after a dog bite. The dog had up-to-date immunizations, and the bite occurred after the boy provoked the attack. Past medical history is unremarkable. He has no known allergies.

Physical Examination: Temperature 38.8°; pulse 120; respirations 14; blood pressure 120/70. General: moderately ill-appearing. HEENT: unremarkable. Neck: supple. Cardiac: regular S_1S_2, no murmur. Chest: clear. Abdomen: soft, nontender. Extremities: purulent, draining bite wound on hand with erythematous streaking up the arm.

Laboratory Findings: Hct 40%; WBC 22,000/μl with 80% neutrophils, 10% bands, 10% lymphocytes; platelets 300,000/μl; hemoglobin 15 g/dl.

Question: What diagnosis should be considered?

Diagnosis: *Pasteurella multocida* infection

Discussion: *Pasteurella multocida* is a small, gram-negative coccobacillus that colonizes the nasopharynx and gastrointestinal tract of cats and dogs. *P. multocida* most commonly causes a localized soft tissue infection or cellulitis after an animal bite, but also causes a wide spectrum of disease including bacteremia, pneumonia, tracheobronchitis, and meningitis, bone and joint infection, and abdominal and pelvic infections.

Pasteurella spp. are nonmotile, nonspore-forming, and bipolar-staining. Most human infection is caused by *P. multocida* (also called *P. septica*), *P. canis, P. stomatis,* and *P. dogmatis*, but there are at least 17 species of *Pasteurella* reported. *P. multocida* is found worldwide in both domestic and wild animals. Cats have the highest rate of colonization (50–90%), followed by dogs (50%), swine (50%), and rats (14%). *Pasteurella* spp. also have been isolated from the human upper respiratory tract and sputum in patients with no underlying disease. Most human infections are acquired through animal bites or scratches; however, nonbite animal exposure, usually via the respiratory tract from contact with contaminated cat secretions, can occur—especially in patients with underlying chronic obstructive pulmonary disease, lung cancer, and bronchiectasis. Cat bites carry a higher risk of *Pasteurella* infection because of the higher rate of *Pasteurella* colonization among cats and because cats have sharper teeth that enable them to inflict deeper, more extensive puncture wounds.

Pain, erythema, and swelling usually develop within several hours of the animal bite. Bite wounds are accompanied by lymphangitic spread in about 25% of cases. Serosanguinous drainage from the bite site typically is noted after 24 hours. Systemic symptoms may be present. In about 40% of cases, a local complication such as osteomyelitis, septic arthritis, or tenosynovitis occurs.

Clinical Manifestations of *Pasteurella* Infection

Cellulitus/soft tissue infections
Osteomyelitis
Upper and lower respiratory tract infections
Meningitis
Intra-abdominal infections

A variety of other pathogens found in normal mouth flora of cats and dogs can produce infection in humans. DF-2 (Capnocytophaga) is a gram-negative rod that grows slowly in most laboratory media and can cause septicemia and meningitis. The incubation period is 4–8 days, and 90% of cases have occurred in immunosuppressed individuals or patients with some underlying chronic medical condition, such as alcoholic liver disease or chronic lung disease. Other "bite pathogens" that can cause disease are streptococci, anaerobes, EF4, M5, and staphylococci.

The treatment of choice for *Pasteurella* infections is penicillin; however, because dog and cat bites tend to be polymicrobial, IV ampicillin-sulbactam or oral amoxicillin-clavulanic acid is recommended for additional antistaphylococcal and anaerobic activity. First-generation cephalosporins and erythromycin have poor activity against *P. multocida*. In the penicillin-allergic adult, doxycycline is the alternate therapy. Surgical debridement often is necessary, as well.

The present patient had an infected dog bite wound and lymphangitis caused by *P. multocida*. He was treated with ampicillin-sulbactam and surgical debridement, with good response.

Clinical Pearls

1. First-generation cephalosporins (cephalexin) have poor activity against *Pasteurella multocida*.

2. Other organisms that cause bite infections are the gram-negative rods DF-2 (Capnocytophaga), EF 4, and M5, as well as streptococci and *Staphylococcus aureus*.

3. In the penicillin-allergic adult, doxycycline is the alternative therapy for *P. multocida* infections.

REFERENCES

1. Weber DJ, Wolfson JS, Swartz MN, et al: *Pasteurella multocida* infections: Report of 34 cases and review of the literature. Medicine 1984; 63:133–154.
2. Weber DJ, Hansen AR: Infections resulting from animal bites. Infect Dis Clin North Am 1991; 5:663–680.
3. Goldstein EJC: Bite wounds and infection. Clin Infect Dis 1992; 14:633–640.

PATIENT 27

An 8-year-old girl with lethargy, fever, and confusion
after swimming in fresh water

An 8-year-old girl living in Florida is brought to the emergency department complaining of abrupt onset and 24-hour duration of high fever, headache, nausea, and vomiting. She was in excellent health prior to this illness and enjoys swimming in a fresh-water pond. No one else is ill in the family. Over the last 4 hours, she has become increasingly lethargic. Past medical history is unremarkable. She has no known allergies.

Physical Examination: Temperature 39.8°; pulse 130; respirations 20; blood pressure 110/70. General: acutely ill-appearing, obtunded. HEENT: negative conjunctivitis, negative otitis. Neck: positive nuchal rigidity. Cardiac: regular rhythm, no murmur. Chest: clear. Abdomen: soft, nontender, positive bowel sounds. Neurologic: cranial nerves II–XII grossly intact, no focal findings.

Laboratory Findings: Hct 36%; WBC 20,000/μl with 90% neutrophils, 10% lymphocytes; hemoglobin 12 g/dl. Cerebrospinal fluid (CSF): WBC 2000/μl with 80% neutrophils, 20% lymphocytes; glucose 30 mg/dl; RBC 2000/μl; protein 150 mg/dl. CSF culture and Gram stain: negative.

Question: What is your diagnosis?

Diagnosis: Amebic meningoencephalitis

Discussion: Primary amebic meningoencephalitis is caused by *Naegleria fowleri* and is a rare disease occurring in previously healthy children and adults who have swum in warm, **freshwater lakes or ponds** where this organism proliferates. *N. fowleri* is found worldwide in soil, lake, pond, and river water, but prefers warm temperatures up to 45°C—conditions found primarily in the southern United States. Usually there is a history of diving into the water, and it is presumed that central nervous system invasion by *N. fowleri* occurs through the cribiform plate.

The incubation period is 2–5 days. Patients present with fever, anorexia, nausea, vomiting, meningismus, and change in mental status. Early on, patients may notice changes in taste or smell. Onset usually is abrupt, and most patients rapidly become comatose and die. Examination of CSF reveals a high white blood cell count typically with a predominance of neutrophils, a low glucose, and an elevated protein. The CSF usually is bloody or sanguinopurulent. Gram stain is characteristically negative, but a wet mount of the CSF demonstrates **red blood cells** and **amebic trophozoites.** Amebic trophozoites have been visualized in 14–16 patients with amebic meningoencephalitis; despite therapy, only 4 patients are known to have survived. There is a 95% mortality rate of primary amebic meningoencephalitis. Treatment of choice is amphotericin B.

Granulomatous amebic encephalitis occurs primarily in **immunocompromised** individuals (e.g., patients with acquired immunodeficiency syndrome), has a gradual onset, and presents with focal neurologic lesions. The diagnosis is made by brain biopsy demonstrating *Acanthamoeba* species or *Leptomyxa* ameba. In a series of 15 patients with granulomatous amebic encephalitis, more than 85% presented with mental status abnormalities. Seizures occurred in 66%, and more than half of the patients had fever, headache, and hemiparesis. The incubation period is not known, since fresh water exposure is not associated with this disease; however, acanthamoeba **skin lesions** have been reported to be present on patients for months prior to onset of encephalitis. Biopsy of the skin ulcers, nodules, or abscesses demonstrates **amebic granulomas.** The diagnosis of granulomatous amebic encephalitis usually is made postmortem. There is no known effective therapy. Drugs shown to be active *in vitro* include pentamidine, ketaconazole, miconazole, and neomycin.

Differential Diagnosis of Amebic
Meningoencephalitis

Meningococcal meningitis
Pneumonococcal meningitis
Early tuberculous meningitis
Cryptococcal meningitis
Viral encephalitis
Endocarditis with cerebral emboli

The present patient had primary amebic meningoencephalitis. The Gram stain and culture of the CSF were negative; however, a wet mount demonstrated RBCs and amebic trophozoites. Despite early initiation of amphotericin B, the patient's condition rapidly deteriorated, and she died 3 days later.

Clinical Pearls

1. Early in the course of illness, patients with amebic meningoencephalitis may notice changes in taste or smell.

2. Gram stain of the CSF is negative, but a wet mount reveals amebic trophozoites.

3. The CSF parameters of amebic meningoencephalitis may mimic purulent bacterial meningitis.

4. The CSF in patients with amebic meningoencephalitis is hemorrhagic.

REFERENCES
1. Duma RJ, Rosenblum WI, McGehee RF, et al: Primary amebic meningoencephalitis caused by *Naegleria*: Two new cases, responses to amphotericin B, and a review. Ann Intern Med 1971; 74:923–932.
2. John DT: Primary amebic meningoencephalitis and the biology of *Naegleria fowleri*. Annu Rev Microbiol 1982; 36:101–123.
3. Anzil AP, Chandrakant R, Wrzolek AA, et al: Amebic encephalitis in a patient with AIDS caused by a newly recognized opportunistic pathogen. Arch Pathol Lab Med 1991; 115:21–25.
4. Brown RL: Successful treatment of primary amebic meningoencephalitis. Arch Intern Med 1991; 151:1201–1202.
5. Gordon SM, Steinberg JP, DuPuis MH, et al: Culture isolation of *Acanthamoeba* species and *Leptomyxid* amebas from patients with amebic meningoencephalitis including patients with AIDS. Clin Infect Dis 1992; 15:1024–1030.

PATIENT 28

A 35-year-old man with multiple penile vesicles

A 35-year-old man comes to your office complaining of painful blisters of 1-day duration on his penis, accompanied by low-grade fever and malaise. He has a new girlfriend and denies multiple sexual partners. He is negative for human immunodeficiency virus (HIV). Past medical history is unremarkable. He has no known allergies.

Physical Examination: Temperature 37.2°; pulse 80; respirations 12; blood pressure 120/80. General: no acute distress. HEENT: normal. Cardiac: regular rhythm, no murmur. Chest: clear. Abdomen: soft, nontender, no organomegaly. Genitals: multiple, tender, vesicular lesions on an erythematous base on glans penis; bilateral inguinal adenopathy.

Laboratory Findings: WBC 8000/µl with 40% neutrophils, 60% lymphocytes. Giemsa stain of vesicle scrapings: multinucleated giant cells (see figure).

Question: What is the most likely clinical diagnosis?

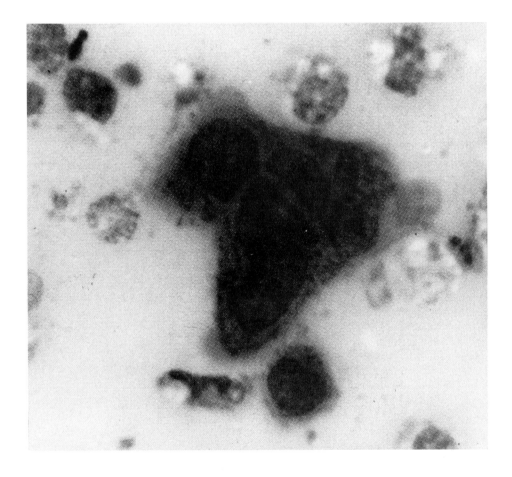

Diagnosis: Primary herpes simplex

Discussion: Primary genital herpes simplex infection usually is caused by herpes simplex virus–type 2 (HSV-2). The incubation period is 2–7 days, and patients present with painful, vesicular lesions that rapidly ulcerate and are accompanied by fever, anorexia, malaise, and inguinal adenopathy. Lesions may appear in a variety of stages, including vesicles, ulcers, and pustules. Lesions are present in the cervix and urethra in more than 80% of women with primary infection.

HSV-1 most commonly causes oral and facial infections, but also can produce genital lesions. Genital infection caused by HSV-1 is much less likely to reactivate than HSV-2 disease. Genital HSV-2 infection recurs up to 10 times more frequently than genital HSV-1 infection. In severe cases, urinary retention from a sacral radiculomyelitis may develop.

Lesions of primary genital herpes tend to be more severe, longer-lasting, and often accompanied by systemic symptoms. Recurrent lesions may be preceded by a prodromal tenderness or burning and tend to heal within 10 days. Primary herpes simplex infection must be distinguished from chancroid, syphilis, erythema multiforme, and local candidiasis.

Severe herpetic infections, including extensive, painful perianal and anal ulcerations as well as herpes proctitis, can occur in HIV-positive patients. *Viral shedding can be asymptomatic, with no active lesions present, in all hosts.* Erythema multiforme may occur following the onset of acute HSV infection, and recurrent attacks of erythema multiforme have been reported. HSV infection may precede up to 75% of cases of erythema multiforme.

The diagnosis of genital HSV infection is made by culturing HSV from the lesions or by demonstrating multinucleated giant cells via Giemsa stain of vesicle base scrapings.

There are now three antiviral agents available for treatment of genital herpes. **Acyclovir** is the only drug available in intravenous form and is therefore the standard treatment for serious HSV infections in both the immunocompetent and immunosuppressed host. **Valacyclovir,** the valyl ester of acyclovir, has greater bioavailability than acyclovir and can be used for treatment and suppression of genital herpes in the normal host. **Famciclovir,** an oral formulation of penciclovir, has similar indications as valacyclovir. Acyclovir, valacyclovir, and famciclovir reduce the duration of the acute infection, speed lesion healing in patients with first episodes of genital herpes, and reduce the frequency or severity or prevent recurrence in 95% of patients taking these medications.

The present patient had primary herpes simplex infection. A scraping of the vesicle base showed multinucleated giant cells, and the viral culture grew HSV-2. He was treated with a 10-day course of oral acyclovir, with resolution of the pain on day 5, and healing of the lesions on day 9.

Clinical Pearls

1. Erythema multiforme may accompany acute HSV infection.
2. Severe genital and perianal HSV infections can occur in patients with acquired immunodeficiency syndrome.
3. Viral shedding may be asymptomatic in patients who have no active lesions.

REFERENCES
1. Mertz GJ: Genital herpes simplex virus infections. Med Clin North Am 1990; 74:1433–1454.
2. Koelle DM, Benedetti J, Langenberg A, et al: Asymptomatic reactivation of herpes simplex virus in women after the first episode of genital herpes. Ann Intern Med 1992; 116:433–438.
3. Whitley RJ, Grann JW; Acyclovir: A decade later. N Engl J Med 1992; 327:782-789.

PATIENT 29

A 10-year-old girl with a lace-like rash on her cheeks

A 10-year-old girl develops a mild fever accompanied by a facial rash. She also complains of sore throat, malaise, and abdominal pain. Several other children in her class have had a similar illness during this spring season.

Physical Examination: Temperature 38°; pulse 90; respirations 14; blood pressure 100/60. General: well-appearing with red cheeks. HEENT: mild pharyngitis; lacey, erythematous, macular rash on cheeks. Cardiac: regular rhythm, no murmur. Chest: clear. Abdomen: soft, nontender, no organomegaly. Extremities: no edema.

Laboratory Findings: Hct 34%; WBC 8000/μl with 65% neutrophils, 5% bands, 30% lymphocytes; platelets 200,000/μl; hemoglobin 12 g/dl.

Question: What condition is the most likely cause of this young girl's symptoms?

Diagnosis: Erythema infectiosum

Discussion: Human parvovirus B19 is a single-stranded DNA virus that causes a number of disorders, including erythema infectiosum, acute arthropathy in adults, a transient aplastic crisis in individuals with chronic hemolytic anemia, and chronic severe anemia in immunocompromised patients. Acute parvovirus infection results in fetal death due to nonimmune fetal hydrops in less than 10% of pregnant women. Most of the severe manifestations of parvovirus B19 infection result from the propensity of the virus to infect and hemolyze erythroid precursors in the bone marrow.

The pathogenesis of B19 infection has been studied in normal human adults. Approximately 1 week after intranasal inoculation, the first phase of a biphasic illness develops. **Phase I** is characterized by viremia of about 1-week duration as well as nonspecific signs and symptoms such as fever, chills, headache, malaise, myalgia, and pruritis. At approximately day 10 of infection, a decrease in reticulocytes accompanied by a mild decrease in hemoglobin is noted on peripheral smear. Examination of the bone marrow demonstrates a marked reduction of erythroid precursors; a mild, transient lymphopenia; neutropenia; and possibly thrombocytopenia. **Phase II** begins about 17 days after nasal inoculation and is characterized by the development of a fine, maculopapular rash accompanied by joint swelling and arthralgia. These symptoms last a few days, mimicking the presentation of erythema infectiosum in adults.

The parvovirus B19–associated rash and arthropathy in the normal host most likely are due to a **self-limited immune complex–mediated disorder.** The normal host tolerates the transient depression of erythropoiesis. However, the patient with hemolytic disease such as sickle cell anemia cannot tolerate the erythroid cell destruction, and acute aplastic crisis results. Immunodeficient patients (e.g., HIV-positive) may be unable to clear B19 viremia, and severe chronic anemia develops.

B19 infections occur worldwide and year round, but most outbreaks occur in school-aged children during the winter and spring months. Transmission probably is via **respiratory secretions.** In school outbreaks, 10–60% of susceptible children develop erythema infectiosum, and the secondary attack rates among susceptible household contacts is about 50%.

B19 also has been transmitted via **contaminated blood** products, especially clotting factor concentrates in hemophiliacs. Patients with transient aplastic crisis are viremic and highly infectious: there has been a case of nosocomial outbreak of B19 among nurses working with these patients. Therefore, pre-

cautions such as private rooms and respiratory and contact isolation methods should be applied.

Clinical manifestations vary depending on the host. The most common presentation in children is erythema infectiosum, also known as fifth disease: a mild, self-limiting, febrile illness accompanied by a "slapped cheek" appearance. The facial rash is lacy or reticular, often mildly pruritic, and also may develop on the arms, legs, trunk, palms, and soles. It lasts for a week, but can recur after exposure to heat, cold, exercise, or water. Sore throat, arthralgia, respiratory symptoms, and mild abdominal pain also can occur. A mild, transient anemia may be present.

Approximately 60% of adults with B19 infection experience **joint involvement,** usually a symmetrical peripheral polyarthropathy involving the hands, knees, or wrists. Approximately 50% of adults have joint involvement without rash. The arthritis lasts 1–2 weeks and typically is self-limited; however, about 5% of adults have symptoms for several months.

Patients with **transient aplastic crisis** caused by B19 infection have underlying chronic hemolytic disease, such as sickle cell disease, thalassemia, hereditary spherocytosis, and autoimmune hemolysis. Patients present with severe anemia and weakness often preceded by a nonspecific prodrome characterized by fever, malaise, and headache. Abdominal complaints and upper respiratory symptoms develop in 30% of children, but rash is uncommon. Generally, the aplastic crisis lasts 1 week, and the bone marrow recovers—but aplastic crisis can cause a life-threatening anemia requiring blood transfusions.

Immunocompromised patients are susceptible to **chronic B19 infection,** resulting in a persistent anemia requiring transfusions. Chronic B19 infection has occurred in patients with AIDS, congenital immunodeficiency, acute lymphocytic leukemia receiving chemotherapy, and bone marrow transplants. Patients present with severe anemia, but rash is uncommon. The treatment of chronic anemia is immunoglobulin therapy, which can control and sometimes cure the disease.

The diagnosis of acute parvovirus B19 infection depends on demonstrating the presence of **IgM antibody.** The virus can be isolated from serum in patients with transient aplastic crisis or chronic anemia, but not in immunocompetent individuals with erythema infectiosum or acute arthropathy. Erythema infectiosum and most cases of acute arthropathy do not require treatment; however, adults with severe arthritis benefit from nonsteroidal anti-inflammatory agents.

In the present patient, facial rash and accompanying symptoms as well as the presence of IgM antibody indicated an acute parvovirus B19 infection. The rash disappeared within 6 days, and full health returned shortly thereafter.

Clinical Pearls

1. Parvovirus B19 infection in adults frequently is accompanied by a symmetrical arthritis.

2. The typical rash of erythema infectiosum has a "slapped cheek" appearance; however, a truncal rash also may be seen.

3. A mild anemia may accompany acute parvovirus B19 infection in normal hosts.

REFERENCES

1. Woolf AD, Campion GV, Chishick A, et al: Clinical manifestations of human parvovirus B19 in adults. Arch Intern Med 1989; 149:1153–1156.
2. Rodis JF, Quinn DL, Gary W, et al: Management and outcomes of pregnancy complicated by human B19 parvovirus infections: A prospective study. Am J Obstet Gynecol 1990; 163:1168–1171.
3. Torok TJ: Parvovirus B19 and human disease. Adv Intern Med 1992; 37:431–455.
4. Serjeant GR, Serjeant BE, Thomas PW, et al: Human parvovirus infection in homozygoces sickle cell disease. Lancet 1993; 1:1237–1240.

PATIENT 30

A 25-year-old Haitian woman with fever and leukopenia

A 25-year-old Haitian woman returns from visiting relatives in Haiti complaining of a 3-day history of fever and shaking chills accompanied by headache, backache, and abdominal pain and followed by profuse sweating. Past medical history is unremarkable. She has no known allergies.

Physical Examination: Temperature 40°; pulse 130; respirations 25; blood pressure 140/80. General: acutely ill-appearing. HEENT: unremarkable. Neck: supple. Cardiac: regular S_1S_2, no murmur. Chest: clear. Abdomen: soft, nontender, without splenomegaly. Extremities: no edema or rash. Neurologic: cranial nerves II–XII grossly intact.

Laboratory Findings: Hct 30%; WBC 3000/μl with 50% neutrophils, 30% bands, 20% lymphocytes; platelets 50,000/μl; hemoglobin 10 g/dl. Chest radiograph: no opacities. Blood cultures: negative, but the laboratory reports intra-erythrocytic parasites (see figure).

Question: How would you diagnose this patient?

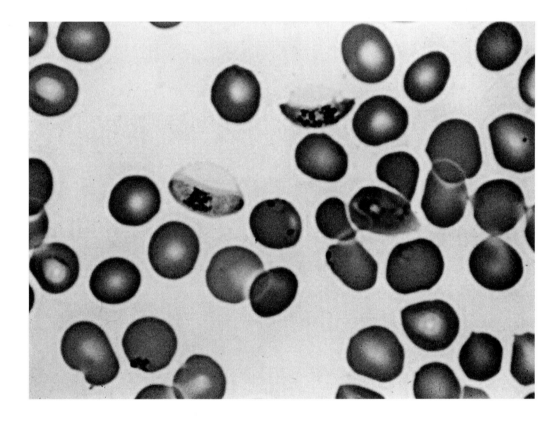

Diagnosis: Malaria (*Plasmodium falciparum*)

Discussion: There are four species of plasmodia causing malaria: *P. falciparum, P. vivax, P. ovale,* and *P. malariae. P. falciparum* causes the most severe disease because it can invade RBC of all ages and can be resistant to many malarial drugs. *P. ovale* and *P. vivax* primarily invade reticulocytes, so the extent of parasitemia is less; however, these species can exist dormant in the liver for prolonged periods of time, resulting in malarial relapses (see table). *P. malariae* can persist in low levels in the blood for decades and can be a cause of transfusion malaria. However, like *P. falciparum, P. malariae* infections do not involve a dormant stage in the liver, and malarial relapse does not occur. The blood smear from a patient with *P. falciparum* malaria shows only ring forms, whereas smears from patients infected with *P. vivax* and *P. ovale* often reveal trophozoites and schizonts. The blood smear of a patient with *P. malariae* shows band or rectangular forms of trophozoites.

The initial symptoms of malaria are nonspecific and mimic a viral syndrome with headache, myalgia, malaise, fever, and chills. Interestingly, classic malarial paroxysms occurring at regular intervals are not often seen in early malaria. The **cyclical fevers** that are the hallmark of malaria occur right before or during the time of red cell lysis, as the schizonts release merozoites into the blood. *P. vivax* and *P. ovale* infections, referred to as tertian malaria, produce a fever spike every 48 hours. *P. malariae* infection (quartan malaria) produces fever every 72 hours. *P. falciparum* infection can produce fever every 48 hours, but an irregular fever pattern is more commonly seen early in disease and in the nonimmune patient.

The typical malarial paroxysm begins with a cold or chilling sensation that lasts from 15 minutes to longer than an hour, during which the patient has **shaking chills.** The second phase is a **"hot stage"** characterized by high fever and sometimes accompanied by tachycardia, hypotension, headache, backache, and abdominal complaints which last several hours. The third phase is the **"sweating stage,"** characterized by marked diaphoresis and resolution of fever.

Laboratory findings in malaria are notable for **leukopenia,** often with a left shift, and **thrombocytopenia.** Mild anemia from hemolysis and splenomegaly may be present. Renal insufficiency can occur from severe *P. falciparum* infection producing proteinuria and hemoglobinuria. The diagnosis of malaria depends on the demonstration of **asexual forms in peripheral blood smears** stained with Wright's or Giemsa stain. Both thin and thick films should be examined. The presence of banana-shaped gametocytes on peripheral smear are diagnostic for *P. falciparum* malaria.

The major, life-threatening complications occurring with severe *P. falciparum* malaria are cerebral malaria, hypoglycemia, renal failure, severe anemia, pulmonary edema, bleeding, disseminated intravascular coagulation, and lactic acidosis. Cerebral malaria is seen most often in children and nonimmune adults. Patients may have a gradual onset of abnormal behavior, confusion, obtundation, or delerium, or the onset may be sudden following a seizure. The onset of coma carries a mortality of 15–20%. Generally, signs of meningeal irritation are absent. Neurologic sequelae occur in 10% of surviving children, but are rare in adults. Hypoglycemia resulting from failure of hepatic gluconeogenesis and increased glucose utilization carries a poor prognosis. Noncardiogenic pulmonary edema is of unclear pathogenesis and is associated with an 80% mortality. Renal failure resembling acute tubular necrosis may require dialysis for several weeks.

Therapy depends on species and severity of disease. Chloroquine is the treatment of choice for *P. vivax, P. ovale,* and *P. malariae,* followed by primaquine phosphate for 14 days for the hepatic phase of *P. vivax* and *P. ovale.* Patients should be tested for G6PD deficiency prior to the administration of primaquine. Severe, resistant *P. falciparum* malaria requires hospitalization and the use of quinidine or quinine combined with tetracycline or pyrimethamine-sulfadoxine. Prevention of malaria depends on avoiding or reducing the frequency of mosquito bites by the use of insect repellants, netting, and proper clothing. Travelers to malarious areas should take antimalarial drug prophylaxis. Chloroquine (once a week) remains the drug of choice for prevention of drug-sensitive *P. falciparum.* However, in many areas of Africa and Asia, there is multi-drug resistant *P. falciparum* malaria, and daily doxycycline or once weekly mefloquine should be used.

The present patient had *P. falciparum* malaria acquired in Haiti, which is sensitive to chloroquine. She received an initial dose of 600 mg chloroquine base orally, followed by a second dose of 300 mg base at 6 hours, and then one dose of 300 mg base daily for 2 days. Her fever and symptoms promptly resolved.

Characteristics of Plasmodia

	P. falciparum	*P. vivax*	*P. ovale*	*P. malariae*
Duration of erythrocytic cycle	48 hours	48 hours	50 hours	72 hours
Type of RBC parasitized	All ages	Reticulocytes	Reticulocytes	Older cells
Morphology	Ring forms, banana shape, gametocytes	Rings, trophozoites, schizonts, Schuffner's dots	Rings, trophozoites, schizonts Schuffner's dots	Trophozoites (band or rectangular shape)
Relapses	No	Yes	Yes	No
Drug resistance	Yes	No	No	No

Clinical Pearls

1. *P. malariae* may persist in the blood for decades and can be a cause of transfusion malaria.

2. Banana-shaped gametocytes on peripheral smear are diagnostic for *P. falciparum* malaria.

3. Malarial relapses occur only with *P. vivax* and *P. ovale,* and treatment requires the addition of primaquine phosphate to eradicate the hepatic phase.

4. Patients should be tested for G6PD deficiency prior to administering primaquine.

REFERENCES
1. Graw GE, Taylor TE, Molyneux ME, et al: Tumor necrosis factor and disease severity in children with falciparum malaria. N Engl J Med 1989; 320:1586–1590.
2. Palmer KJ, Holliday SM, Brogden RN: Mefloquine: A review of its antimalarial activity, pharmacokinetic properties, and therapeutic efficacy. Drugs 1993; 45:430–475.
3. Wyler DJ: Chemoprophylaxis of malaria. N Engl J Med 1993; 329:31–37.
4. White NJ: The treatment of malaria. N Engl J Med 1996; 335:800–806.

PATIENT 31

An 18-year-old college student with cough, conjunctivitis, and macular eruption

An 18-year-old college student complains of fever, cough, conjunctivitis, and a diffuse red rash that began on her face and then progressed downward to involve her neck and extremities. She also complains of rhinorrhea. Past medical history is unremarkable.

Physical Examination: Temperature 38.8°; pulse 120; respirations 18; blood pressure 130/80. General: ill-appearing, with conjunctival suffusion and diffuse rash. HEENT: positive conjunctivitis, gray specks on buccal mucosa. Neck: supple. Cardiac: regular rhythm, no murmur. Chest: clear. Abdomen: soft, nontender, no organomegaly. Skin: diffuse, erythematous, maculopapular rash (see figure).

Laboratory Findings: Hct 38%; WBC 6000/μl with 40% neutrophils, 60% lymphocytes; platelets 300,000/μl.

Question: What is the most likely clinical diagnosis?

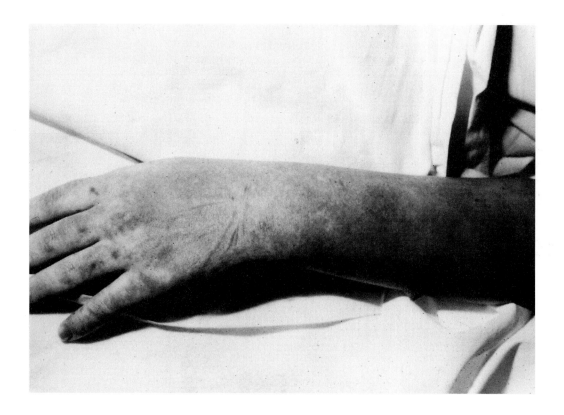

Diagnosis: Measles

Discussion: Measles is a highly contagious viral disease caused by the rubeola virus. The incubation period is 10–14 days. It is spread via airborne respiratory secretions and contracted by direct contact with infected respiratory droplets. Patients are infectious during the late prodrome phase of illness, from approximately 2 days prior to the onset of rash until 4 days after its appearance. The prodromal phase lasts several days and begins with malaise, fever, cough, coryza, and conjunctivitis.

Koplik spots consisting of bluish-gray specks resembling grains of sand may be seen on the buccal mucosa just before the appearance of the rash. The presence of Koplik spots is pathognomonic of measles. The rash in measles is maculopapular and nonpruritic, and it begins on the face and then moves downward to involve the neck, chest, and extremities—including the palms and soles. The rash may desquamate with healing. Fever usually resolves by the fourth or fifth day of rash. Lymphadenopathy, splenomegaly, and gastrointestinal complaints also may be present. Laboratory findings are notable for leukopenia and lymphopenia.

The major complications of measles are **pneumonia** and **encephalitis.** The measles virus has a great propensity to invade the respiratory tract. Chest films often are abnormal even in uncomplicated cases. Pneumonia may be due to direct viral invasion or bacterial superinfection, usually by pneumococci, streptococci, staphylococci or *Haemophilus.* Viral invasion of the central nervous system is common, and up to 50% of patients without neurologic findings will have abnormal electroencephalography. However, only 1 in 2000 patients develops acute measles encephalitis. Patients with this complication present with headache, seizures, drowsiness, and coma, usually several days after the onset of rash. Acute encephalitis appears to be an immune-mediated response to myelin proteins, rather than direct viral invasion of the brain. The clinical course of acute measles encephalitis varies from mild to severe, with residual neurologic sequelae. Subacute sclerosing panencephalitis, a rare, chronic measles encephalitis that results in progressive dementia, has been almost completely eliminated by measles vaccination.

The diagnosis of measles is based primarily on clinical findings of cough, coryza, conjunctivitis, Koplik spots, and the characteristic rash. Laboratory diagnosis is made by demonstrating a fourfold rise in measles antibody titer in acute and convalescent serum or a positive ELISA IgM antibody, or by immunofluorescent staining of a smear of respiratory secretions for measles antigen.

Atypical measles is a syndrome that has occurred in persons who received the killed measles vaccine, which is no longer administered. In atypical measles, the rash begins peripherally and often appears vesicular or urticarial in nature. It often is accompanied by high fevers, pulmonary opacities, and hepatitis. The diagnosis of atypical measles is made on the basis of the characteristic clinical course accompanied by the production of high measles antibody titers.

Measles in patients with defects in cell-mediated immunity can be particularly severe or fatal. Giant-cell pneumonia and progressive encephalitis are common complications. Tuberculosis can be aggravated in patients who develop measles. The tuberculin test may become negative after measles or measles vaccination due to depression of cell-mediated immunity by measles virus.

Prevention of measles depends on administering two doses of live measles vaccine (usually combined with mumps and rubella) to children at age 12–15 months, and then on entry into school at age 4–6 years. Administration of gamma globulin shortly after exposure can alter the course of disease in immunosuppressed patients. Gamma globulin may prolong the incubation period for up to 20 days and shorten the prodromal phase. It reduces the severity of fever, rash, respiratory symptoms, and conjunctivitis.

The present patient had a classic case of measles, with fever, cough, conjunctivitis, and coryza. The findings of Koplik spots and a maculopapular rash beginning on the face and then proceeding down the body confirmed the diagnosis. The patient did well without treatment, and fever and rash resolved by day 5.

Clinical Pearls

1. Patients are infectious during the late prodromal phase (about 2 days prior to rash) and about 4 days after the appearance of the rash.

2. Koplik spots are pathognomonic of measles.

3. Atypical measles is a syndrome described in persons receiving the killed measles vaccine. It is characterized by a rash beginning peripherally and often is accompanied by pneumonia, hepatitis, high fever, and the production of high measles antibody titers.

4. The tuberculin test may become negative after measles or measles vaccination due to depression of cell-mediated immunity by measles virus.

REFERENCES

1. Annunziato D, Kaplan M, Hall WW, et al: Atypical measles syndrome: Pathologic and serologic features. Pediatrics 1982; 70:203–209.
2. Krasinski K, Borkowsky W: Measles and measles immunity in children infected with human immunodeficiency virus. JAMA 1989; 261:2512–2516.
3. Gindler JS, Atkinson W, Markowitz LE, et al: Epidemiology of measles in the United States in 1989 and 1990. Pediatr Infect Dis J 1992; 11:841–846.
4. Kaplan LJ, Daum RS, Smaron M, et al: Severe measles in immunocompromised patients. JAMA 1992; 267:1237–1241.

PATIENT 32

A 20-year-old man with a painful lump in his neck
2 weeks after a tooth extraction

A 20-year-old man comes to the emergency department complaining of fever and a lump in his neck that he noticed 1 week prior. The lump is not painful, but he noted drainage from his neck and has had daily fever to 38.6°C. He has been undergoing extensive dental work over the last 2 months and had a tooth extraction 2 weeks ago.

Physical Examination: Temperature 38.6°; pulse 110; respirations 12; blood pressure 140/80. General: moderate distress, with a swollen jaw. Mouth: nontender submandibular mass, small amount of purulent drainage with granules. Neck: supple. Cardiac: normal. Chest: clear. Abdomen: soft, nontender, normal bowel sounds. Extremities: no edema.

Laboratory Findings: WBC 20,000/μl with 75% polymorphonuclear cells, 5% bands, 20% lymphocytes. Gram stain of neck drainage: filamentous, gram-positive rods (see figure).

Question: What is the most likely cause of the patient's medical presentation?

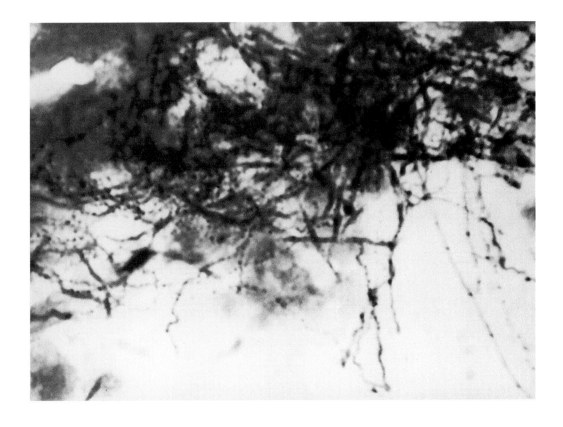

Diagnosis: Actinomycosis

Discussion: Actinomyces israelli, a gram-positive anaerobic rod, is the most frequently isolated agent causing actinomycosis. Oral-cervicofacial actinomycosis, or **"lumpy jaw,"** is the most common form. Patients present with a slowly enlarging, painless soft-tissue mass at the angle of the jaw that has developed after dental work or trauma. Without treatment the disease spreads across tissue planes, and characteristic **sinus tracts**—discharging tiny, actinomycotic sulfur granules—may develop in the skin. Besides the submandibular location, cervicofacial actinomycosis can involve the maxilla, sinuses, external ear, temporal bone, and lacrimal glands. Thoracic, abdominal and pelvic actinomycosis also are common. Intra-abdominal actinomycosis usually is secondary to abdominal perforation from other causes. Pelvic actinomycosis also may develop from intra-abdominal infection, but more often is associated with the presence of intrauterine contraceptive devices (IUDs). Infection associated with IUDs can result in endometritis, hydronephrosis, rectal involvement, or extension to the abdominal wall.

The diagnosis of actinomycosis is made histologically by identifying the **sulfur granules,** which consist of colonies of *Actinomyces* surrounded by inflammatory cells, in tissue or sterile fluid. Cultures must be incubated anaerobically, are difficult to grow, and often are negative—especially if the patient received prior antibiotics. Actinomycosis must be distinguished from nocardiosis and botryomycosis by culture and biopsy.

The treatment of choice is high-dose **penicillin** given intravenously for 6 weeks followed by oral penicillin for 6–12 months. Surgical drainage of abscesses as well as resection of chronic sinus tracts may be necessary. In the penicillin-allergic patient, doxycycline has been used in the treatment of cervicofacial actinomycosis; however, it is contraindicated in children under 8 years of age and in pregnant women. Alternative antibiotics include clindamycin and erythromcyin.

The present patient exhibited filamentous, gram-positive *A. israelli* on Gram stain of the neck drainage. He was treated with 24 million units of intravenous penicillin G for 6 weeks, followed by oral phenoxymethyl penicillin for another 10 months, until all evidence of active infection had resolved.

Clinical Pearls

1. Actinomycosis is characterized by the appearance of multiple, draining sinus tracts.

2. The sulphur granule is composed of colonies of *Actinomyces* surrounded by inflammatory cells.

3. Actinomycosis must be distinguished from nocardiosis and botryomycosis by culture and biopsy.

REFERENCES

1. Bennhoff D: Actinomycosis: Diagnostic and therapeutic considerations and a review of 32 cases. Laryngoscope 1984; 94:1198–1217.
2. Lerner PI: The lumpy jaw: Cervicofacial actinomycosis. Infect Dis Clin North Am 1988; 2:203–220.
3. Burden P: Actinomycosis. J Infect 1989; 19:95–99.

PATIENT 33

A 40-year-old HIV-positive man with headache and fever

A 40-year-old man comes to the emergency department complaining of a 2-week history of fever and headache. He is HIV-positive with a CD_4 count of 80/μl. His current medications are zidovudine, lamivudine, and indinavir, as well as prophylactic trimethoprim-sulfamethoxazole. He denies dyspnea. diarrhea, nausea, vomiting, and confusion. Past medical history is significant for *Pneumocystis carinii* pneumonia 1 year prior. He has no known allergies.

Physical Examination: Temperature 38.6°; pulse 100; respirations 14; blood pressure 110/70. General: cachectic, moderate distress. HEENT: oral thrush. Neck: nuchal rigidity. Cardiac: regular rate, no murmur. Abdomen: soft, nontender. Chest: clear. Neurologic: cranial nerves intact. Skin: no lesions.

Laboratory Findings: Hct 26%; WBC 2500/μl with 90% polymorphonuclear cells, 10% lymphocytes; platelets 150,000/μl. Cerebrospinal fluid: 600 nucleated cells with 80% lymphocytes, 20% polymorphonuclear cells; glucose 10 mg/dl; protein 150 mg/dl. Gram stain: negative. India ink: see figure.

Questions: What is your diagnosis? What treatment would you begin?

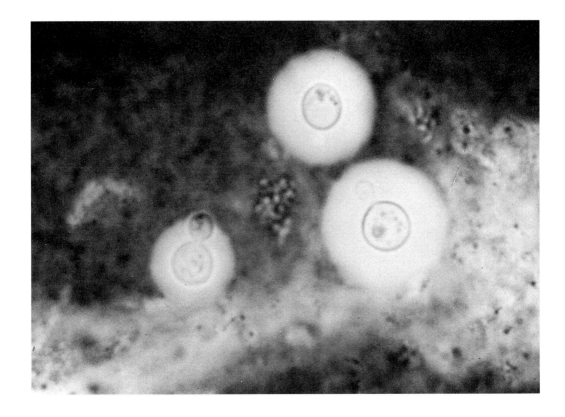

Diagnosis: Cryptococcal meningitis

Discussion: *Cryptococcus neoformans* is an encapsulated, yeast-like fungus that is the cause of cryptococcosis. Most patients in whom invasive cryptococcal disease develops are immunosuppressed; however, cases have occurred in normal hosts. The lung is the portal of entry for cryptococcus, although cryptococcal pneumonia occurs in less than 15% of infected patients. The most common and most severe form of disease is cryptococcal meningitis.

Cryptococcal meningitis occurs primarily in immunocompromised patients, especially in those with AIDs, but also in patients with lymphomas, transplantations, and long-term, high-dose steroid regimens. Approximately 10% of patients with AIDS acquire cryptococcal disease when their CD_4 count falls below 200/μl. Cryptococcal meningitis may have an acute or gradual onset. Patients typically complain of headache, fever, and malaise of 1- to 2-week duration; some patients also experience confusion, nausea, vomiting, lethargy, and behavioral changes. Patients may demonstrate impaired memory, cranial nerve involvement, and seizures. Note, however, that some HIV-positive patients have minimal or no symptoms. Physical examination is notable for papilledema in up to 30% and cranial nerve palsies in 20%. Nuchal rigidity usually is absent. A CT scan or MRI of the brain demonstrates a concomitant cryptococcoma in 30% of patients with cryptococcal meningitis.

Cerebrospinal fluid (CSF) almost always is abnormal, with a lymphocytic pleocytosis, elevated protein, depressed glucose, and elevated opening pressure. **India ink smears** are positive in 50–90% of cases, and **CSF cryptococcal polysaccharide capsular antigen** is positive in more than 90%. In addition, *Cryptococcal neoformans* can be cultured from the CSF and sometimes from the blood.

A number of laboratory findings predict a poor prognosis: elevated opening pressure, positive India ink preparation, high titer of cryptococcal antigen in CSF or blood, hypoglycorrhachia, and a poor inflammatory response manifested by few lymphocytes in the CSF. Some AIDS patients with overwhelming cryptococcal meningitis may have a normal CSF cell count and glucose, but the India ink preparation and cryptococcal antigen almost always are positive.

Cryptococcosis can involve a number of other sites outside the central nervous system. **Pulmonary cryptococcosis** may be asymptomatic or may cause bilateral pneumonia in HIV-positive patients. Pulmonary cryptococcosis may occur alone or accompany cryptococcosis in the central nervous system. Forty percent of patients with pulmonary cryptococcosis have chest pain, and approximately 20% present with cough and dyspnea.

Cutaneous cryptococcosis is seen in 10% of patients with cryptococcosis. The lesions appear as small papules, pustules, or ulcers and usually are asymptomatic. In AIDS patients, lesions appear as umbilicated papules resembling the lesions of molluscum contagiosum. Other, less common manifestations of cryptococcosis include bone disease, prostatitis, chorioretinitis, endocarditis, sinusitis, hepatitis, and renal abscess.

The standard treatment of cryptococcal meningitis and other serious cryptococcosis is **amphotericin B,** either high-dose (0.6 mg/kg/day) alone, or low-dose (0.3 mg/kg/day) plus flucytosine. Non-AIDS patients should be treated for a 6-week course. Patients with AIDS require life-long suppressive therapy. Importantly, **fluconazole** has been shown as effective as amphotericin B in patients with AIDS.

In the present patient, the CSF cryptococcal antigen was positive at 1:64. He was begun on amphotericin B, 0.6 mg/kg/day for 2 weeks, and then changed to oral fluconazole, 400 mg daily, for maintenance therapy for an indefinite period of time. His headache and fever resolved over a 2-week period.

Clinical Pearls

1. In AIDS patients with overwhelming cryptococcal meningitis, CSF cell count and glucose may be normal, but the India ink and cryptococcal antigen almost always are positive.

2. Cryptococcal meningitis in patients with AIDS may be treated with either fluconazole or amphotericin B.

3. Poor prognostic factors for cryptococcal meningitis are: an elevated opening pressure, low CSF glucose level, a CSF nucleated cell count $< 20/\mu l$, a positive India ink preparation, positive blood cultures, and a high cryptococcal antigen titer.

REFERENCES

1. Larsen RA, Leal MAE, Chan LS: Fluconazole compared with amphotericin B plus flucytosine for cryptococcal meningitis in AIDS: A randomized trial. Ann Intern Med 1990; 113:183–187.
2. Powderly WG: Therapy for cryptococcal meningitis in patients with AIDS. Clin Infect Dis 1992; 14(suppl 1): 554–559.
3. White M, Cirrincione C, Blevins A, Armstrong D: Cryptococcal meningitis: Outcome in patients with AIDS and patients with neoplastic disease. Clin Infect Dis 1992; 165:960–963.

PATIENT 34

A 20-year-old man with a generalized maculopapular eruption on the palms

A 20-year-old man complains of a diffuse, erythematous rash; malaise; and low-grade temperature. The rash is not pruritic. The patient denies headache, stiff neck, sore throat, diarrhea, and urethral discharge. All childhood immunizations have been received. The patient is sexually active. Past medical history is unremarkable, and there are no known allergies.

Physical Examination: Temperature 37°; pulse 80; respirations 14; blood pressure 110/70. General: no apparent distress. HEENT: no pharyngitis. Neck: supple. Cardiac: regular S_1S_2, no murmur. Chest: clear. Abdomen: soft, nontender, no organomegaly. Skin: diffuse, erythematous, maculopapular rash involving palms and soles (see figure). Genitals: no lesions.

Laboratory Findings: WBC 15,000/μl with 60% polymorphonuclear cells, 5% bands, 20% lymphocytes. Alkaline phosphatase 400 IU/L, alanine aminotransferase 40 IU/L, aspartate aminotransferase 100 IU/L.

Question: What is the likely diagnosis?

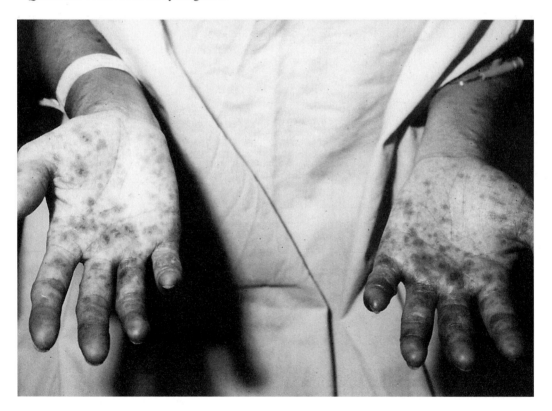

Diagnosis: Secondary syphilis

Discussion: Syphilis is a sexually transmitted, systemic infection caused by *Treponema pallidum*. The primary lesion is a painless chancre that appears at the site of inoculation approximately 3 weeks after infection. Characteristically, it has an indurated appearance and heals spontaneously. Secondary syphilis usually occurs 6–8 weeks after healing of the chancre and typically is manifested by the presence of a diffuse, symmetrical rash on the palms and soles. The rash of secondary syphilis can be macular, papular, maculopapular, or pustular, but never vesicular. It can have a psoriatic appearance, especially in HIV-positive individuals. A variety of other physical symptoms may occur, including patchy alopecia; mucous patches on the lips, tongue, or oral mucosa; condylomata; generalized lymphadenopathy; and constitutional symptoms such as fever, weight loss, malaise, and headache. Syphilitic hepatitis (characterized by an elevated alkaline phosphatase), renal involvement, anterior uveitis, and acute meningitis also can occur. Untreated syphilis can progress to latent and late syphilis.

The diagnosis of primary syphilis is made by a positive darkfield examination of the chancre. The diagnosis of secondary syphilis usually is made by serology. The rapid plasmin reagin (RPR) and the Veneral Disease Research Laboratory (VDRL) test are **nontreponemal antibody tests** that are close to 100% positive in secondary syphilis. The titers of these serologic tests decrease after appropriate therapy; therefore, they are useful in assessing adequacy of therapy. The fluorescent treponemal antibody–absorbed (FTA-ABS) and microhemagglutination-*Treponema pallidum* (MHA-TP) are the standard **treponemal antibody tests**. They are very specific and confirm a positive VDRL or RPR; however, the FTA-ABS and MHA-TP remain positive after therapy. False positive serologic tests for syphilis can occur in drug addiction, systemic lupus erythematosus, viral infection in the elderly, hypergammaglobulinemia, and a variety of infectious diseases, as well as after vaccination (see table).

Infectious Diseases Causing False Positive Serologic Tests

Lyme disease	HIV infection
Tuberculosis	Epstein-Barr infection
Leptospirosis	Malaria
Mycoplasma	Endocarditis
pneumonia	Pneumococcal
Varicella	pneumonia
Hepatitis	

Treatment of choice remains **benzathine penicillin** 2.4 million units in a single dose for primary or secondary syphilis in a normal host. Latent or late syphilis requires three weekly injections of 2.4 million units of benzathine penicillin. Neurosyphilis is treated with 10 days of intravenous high-dose penicillin G. Patients who are HIV-positive may require multiple injections, close follow up to detect relapses, and lumbar puncture to exclude syphilis.

The present patient had an RPR of 1:64 and a positive FTA-ABS. He was treated with a single injection of 2.4 million units of benzathine penicillin. An HIV test was negative. Repeat serologic testing every 3 months showed a declining RPR titer, which reverted to negative 1 year later.

Clinical Pearls

1. The rash of secondary syphilis can be macular, maculopapular, papular, or pustular, but never vesicular.

2. The rash of secondary syphilis can resemble psoriasis in HIV-positive patients.

3. False-positive serologic tests for syphilis can occur in drug addiction, collagen vascular disease (especially systemic lupus erythematosus), viral infections in the elderly, hypergammaglobulinemia, and in a variety of infectious diseases, as well as after vaccination.

REFERENCES

1. Romanowski B, Sutherland R, Fick GH, et al: Serologic response to treatment of infectious syphilis. Ann Intern Med 1991; 114:1005–1009.
2. Hook EW III, Marra C: Acquired syphilis in adults. N Engl J Med 1992; 326:1060–1069.
3. Musher DM, Hamill RJ, Baughm RE: Effect of human immunodeficiency virus (HIV) infection on the course of syphilis and on the response to treatment. Ann Intern Med 1992; 113:872–881.
4. Jurado RL: Syphilis serology: A practical approach. Inf Dis Clin Practice 1996; 5:351–358.

PATIENT 35

A 30-year-old man with painful, warm, spreading cellulitis of the leg

A 30-year-old man comes to the emergency department complaining of a painful right leg. Two days earlier he was bitten by an insect on his lower leg. The next day he noted redness and swelling around the bite, and these symptoms rapidly spread up his leg. His past medical history is unremarkable, and he has no known allergies.

Physical Examination: Temperature 39.4°; pulse 120; respirations 12; blood pressure 130/80. General: moderate distress. HEENT: no pharyngitis. Neck: supple. Cardiac: no murmur. Abdomen: soft, nontender, normal bowel sounds. Extremities: erythematous right leg, swollen and tender (see figure).

Laboratory Findings: Hct 36%; WBC 21,000/μl with granulocytes 80%, bands 10%; lymphocytes 10%; platelets 250,000/μl.

Question: What condition is suggested by the patient's clinical presentation?

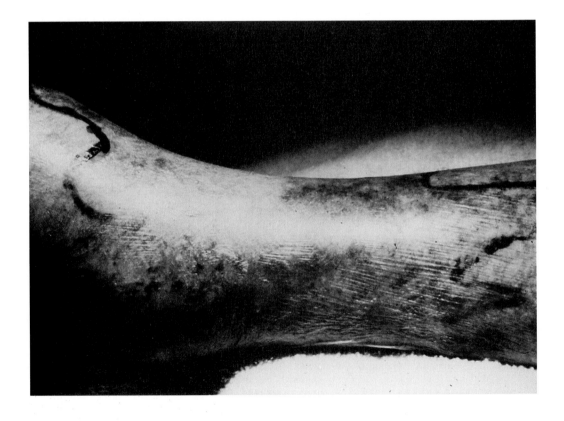

Diagnosis: Group A streptococcal cellulitis

Discussion: The group A streptococcus is a common cause of infections of the skin and soft tissues, especially impetigo, erysipelas, lymphangitis, and cellulitis. Streptococcal cellulitis is a **rapidly spreading inflammation** of the skin and subcutaneous tissues, usually occurring after trauma (sometimes mild or inapparent) or surgery. The patient develops fever, chills, malaise, local pain, erythema, and swelling, and there is a superficial desquamation of the skin overlying the area of cellulitis. Blood cultures may be positive for *S. pyogenes.*

Streptococcal cellulitis may be complicated by streptococcal toxic shock syndrome (TSS). Patients with streptococcal TSS most often have invasive soft tissue infections, rapidly developing hypotension, multiorgan failure, and sunburn-like macular rash. Most patients with streptococcal TSS are previously healthy individuals. Some cases have occurred in children due to secondary infection of varicella lesions with group A streptococcus.

Recurrent group A streptococcal cellulitis has occurred in patients with impaired lymphatic drainage. Women who have undergone a radical mastectomy are at risk for recurrent arm cellulitis. Recurrent leg cellulitis has developed in patients after coronary bypass surgery in the leg from which the saphenous vein was removed, especially in the presence of tinea pedis. Streptococci presumably gain entrance into the extremity through the small abrasions between the toes. Therapy involves treatment of the streptococcal infection as well as topical antifungal for the tinea pedis. Parenteral drug abusers also have an increased risk of streptococcal cellulitis, often associated with bacteremia, endocarditis, or septic thrombophlebitis.

Penicillin is the drug of choice for streptococcal cellulitis; however, cephalosporins providing broader coverage are a good choice for empiric therapy. In the penicillin-allergic patient, vancomycin or clindamycin are preferred.

The present patient was suspected to have streptococcal cellulitis of the leg on the basis of the bite history, rapid spread of erythema, and fever. Demonstration of *S. pyogenes* on blood culture confirmed the diagnosis. He was treated with cefazolin, 1 g intravenously every 8 hours, with prompt defervescence of his fever and rapid improvement of cellulitis over the next 7 days.

Clinical Pearls

1. Patients with impaired lymphatic drainage may have recurrent cellulitis.

2. Recurrent streptococcal leg cellulitis may occur in patients after coronary bypass surgery if the saphenous vein was removed.

3. Parenteral drug abusers have an increased risk of streptococcal cellulitis often associated with bacteremia, endocarditis, or septic thrombophlebitis.

REFERENCES

1. Stevens DL, Tanner MH, Winship J, et al: Severe group A streptococcal infections associated with a toxic shock-like syndrome and scarlet fever toxin. N Engl J Med 1989; 321:1–7.
2. Stevens DL: Invasive group A streptococcal infections. Clin Infect Dis 1991; 14:2–13.
3. Hoge CW, Schwartz B, Talkington DF, et al: The changing epidemiology of invasive group A streptococcal infections and the emergence of streptococcal toxic shock-like symptoms: A retrospective population-based study. JAMA 1993; 269:384–389.

PATIENT 36

A 58-year-old woman with fever, fatigue, and heart murmur

A 58-year-old woman complained of a 2-week history of low-grade fever, malaise, fatigue, and anorexia. Three weeks ago she underwent a routine dental cleaning. She denied cough, headache, and abdominal pain.

Physical Examination: Temperature 38.8°; pulse 90; respirations 22; blood pressure 130/70. General: mildly ill appearance. HEENT: Conjunctival petechiae (see figure). Chest: clear. Cardiac: regular rate, grade II/VI systolic murmur radiating to apex. Abdomen: soft, nontender, no organomegaly. Extremities: splinter hemorrhages on fingernails; erythematous, painless macule on palm.

Laboratory Findings: WBC 15,000/μl with 75% neutrophils, 7% bands, 15% lymphocytes, 3% monocytes. Urinalysis: WBC 20/hpf, RBC 5/hpf, 2+ protein. Blood cultures: two sets growing gram-positive cocci in chains.

Question: What diagnosis can explain this patient's clinical condition?

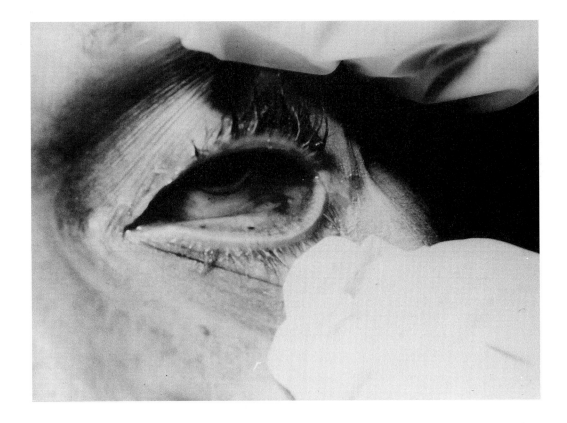

Diagnosis: *Streptococcal viridans* endocarditis

Discussion: Endocarditis, an infection of the endocardium that usually involves a heart valve, occurs in three settings: native valve, prosthetic valve, and intravenous drug use. **Native valve endocarditis** is most commonly caused by streptococci, enterococci, and staphylococci. Streptococci are the etiologic agent in approximately 55% of cases of native valve endocarditis, and viridans streptococci, which are part of the normal oropharyngeal flora, cause 75% of the cases of streptococcal endocarditis. Staphylococci account for about 30% of native valve infections, and enterococci about 6%. A number of other bacteria, including the HACEK group (*Hemophilus, Actinobacillus, Cardiobacterium, Eikenella,* and *Kingella*), *Pneumococcus, Neisseria, Escherichia coli,* and other gram-negatives, are occasional causes of native valve endocarditis.

Approximately 70% of patients with native valve endocarditis have an abnormality of the cardiac valve such as rheumatic valvular disease, congenital heart disease, mitral valve prolapse, or degenerative/calcific disease.

In contrast, *Staphylococcus aureus* causes more than 50% of cases of **endocarditis in intravenous drug users,** followed by streptococci and enterococci (20%), *Candida* (6%), and gram-negative bacilli (6%). The most common causes of early **prosthetic valve endocarditis** are *S. epidermidis* and *S. aureus* (50%), followed by gram-negative bacilli (15%), and fungi (10%). The most common causes of late prosthetic valve endocarditis are streptococci (40%) and staphylococci (30%).

Culture-negative endocarditis comprises less than 5% of cases and is usually due to fastidious bacteria such as *Hemophilus* spp., *Brucella, Bacteroides,* nutritionally deficient streptococci, *Chlamydia,* and *Coxiella burnetii.*

The symptoms of endocarditis are nonspecific. Patients with *Streptococcus viridans* endocarditis generally have a subacute presentation, with low grade fever, malaise, and arthralgia. Almost all patients have an audible heart murmur. A number of other physical findings such as petechiae, splenomegaly, splinter hemorrhages, Roth spots (retinal hemorrhages with clear center), Osler nodes (small, tender nodules on fingers or toes), Janeway lesions (painless macules on palms and soles), and clubbing may be seen. A third of patients experience embolic events such as cerebral emboli, renal emboli, or emboli to large arteries of the extremities. Embolic events may occur even after starting antimicrobial therapy.

Fungal endocarditis, in particular, often is complicated by large, peripheral emboli. Persistent fever after 1 week of appropriate antimicrobial therapy may signify the presence of metastatic abscesses, especially a splenic abscess. Other complications of endocarditis include mycotic aneurysms, myocardial abscess, meningitis, brain abscess, congestive heart failure due to valvular destruction, and coronary artery emboli.

Anemia (normocytic normochromic) usually is present, and proteinuria and hematuria occur in most patients. Blood cultures are positive in over 95% of patients. A transthoracic echocardiogram demonstrates vegetations in 50–80% of cases, and transesophageal echocardiograms are positive in over 90% of cases.

Penicillin-susceptible (minimal inhibitory concentration [MIC] $\leq$ 0.1 μg/nl) *S. viridans* endocarditis can be treated with 4 weeks of penicillin G, 12–18 million units per day, or ceftriaxone, 2g (IV) once daily. A short-course therapy of 2 weeks of penicillin G combined with gentamicin or streptomycin for faster bacteriocidal effect is an alternative regimen. Four weeks of intravenous vancomycin therapy can be used in β-lactam-allergic patients. A 4-week course of penicillin with an aminoglycoside for the first 2 weeks is effective in patients with endocarditis due to viridans streptococci with penicillin MIC $\geq$ 0.1 μg/ml and in patients with nutritionally deficient streptococci.

Indications for valve replacement include intractable heart failure, inability to eradicate infection, fungal endocarditis, myocardial abscess, and multiple embolic events.

The present patient exhibited an audible heart murmur, petechiae, and splinter hemorrhages. Gram-positive cocci in her blood cultures were identified as *S. viridans.* The diagnosis was confirmed by a transesophageal echocardiogram revealing a mitral valve vegetation, moderate mitral regurgitation, and a prolapsed mitral valve. She was begun on ceftriaxone, 2 g IV each day, and she defervesced on day 3 of antimicrobial therapy. Repeat blood cultures were negative, and the patient completed a 4-week course of ceftriaxone.

Clinical Pearls

1. Streptococci cause 55% of all cases of native valve endocarditis in patients who do not abuse intravenous drugs.

2. Culture-negative endocarditis comprises less than 5% of cases and is usually due to fastidious bacteria such as *Hemophilus* spp., *Brucella, Bacteroides,* nutritionally deficient streptococci, *Chlamydia,* and *Coxiella burnetii.*

3. Fungal endocarditis often is complicated by large peripheral emboli.

4. Metastatic abscesses (especially a splenic abscess) should be considered in a patient who continues febrile after 1 week of appropriate antimicrobial therapy.

REFERENCES

1. Roberts RB, Kreiger AG, Schiller NI, et al: Viridans streptococcal endocarditis: The role of various species including pyridoxal-dependent streptococci. Rev Infect Dis 1979; 1:955–965.
2. Sussman JI, Baron EJ, Tenebaum MJ, et al: Viridans streptococcal endocarditis: Clinical, microbiological, and echocardiographic correlations. J Infect Dis 1986; 154:597–603.
3. Murphy JG, Foster-Smith K: Management of complications of infective endocarditis with emphasis on echocardiographic findings. Infect Dis Clin North Am 1993; 7:153–165.
4. Wilson WR, Karchmer AW, Dajani AS, et al: Antibiotic treatment of adults with infective endocarditis due to streptococci, enterococci, staphylococci, and HACEK microorganisms. JAMA 1995; 274:1706–1713.

PATIENT 37

An 18-year-old woman with fever, pharyngitis, and macular eruption

An 18-year-old woman complains of fever, sore throat, malaise, and generalized erythematous rash. Her sister recently was treated with penicillin for a sore throat. Past medical history is unremarkable. She has no known allergies.

Physical Examination: Temperature 38.8°; pulse 120; respirations 14; blood pressure 120/70. General: uncomfortable appearing, no acute distress. HEENT: exudative pharyngitis, "strawberry" tongue. Neck: supple. Cardiac: S_1S_2 normal, no organomegaly. Extremities: no edema. Skin: diffuse, erythematous, sandpaper-like rash (see figure).

Laboratory Findings: Hct 36%; WBC 20,000/μl with 80% neutrophils, 10% bands, 10% lymphocytes; platelets 200,000/μl. Gram stain of throat: polymorphonuclear cells and gram-positive cocci in chains.

Question: What is your diagnosis?

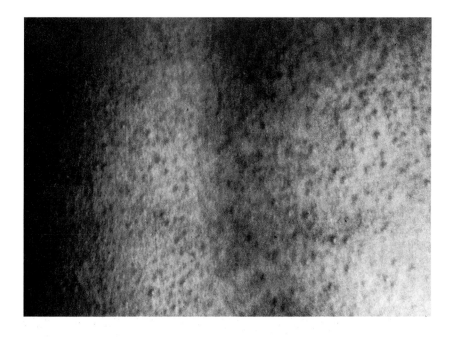

Diagnosis: Scarlet fever

Discussion: *Streptococcus pyogenes* (group A streptococci) is the most frequent bacterial cause of acute pharyngitis and a common cause of skin and soft tissue infection. Group A streptococcal pharyngitis occurs primarily in school-aged children 5–15 years old; however, all age groups are susceptible. The disease is spread from person to person via droplets of saliva or nasal secretions. Crowding facilitates the spread of group A streptococci, and epidemics of acute streptococcal pharyngitis have occurred in the military. Some individuals become colonized with group A streptococci. Several studies have shown a 15–20% pharyngeal carriage rate among school-aged children, especially among family contacts of patients with streptococcal pharyngitis.

The incubation period of streptococcal pharyngitis is 2–4 days. Patients present with an acute onset of sore throat accompanied by fever, malaise, and headache. Children may complain of gastrointestinal discomfort. On examination, the pharynx is erythematous and the tonsils are enlarged, hyperemic, and coated with a **white exudate.** Cervical adenopathy usually is present. Rhinorrhea, coryza, hoarseness, and cough are rarely seen with streptococcal pharyngitis, although they commonly accompany viral pharyngitis. Laboratory findings include leukocytosis, positive throat culture for group A streptococcus, and positive c-reactive protein.

Scarlet fever most often occurs after pharyngeal infection with a group A streptococcus that produces pyrogenic exotoxin (erythrogenic toxin). It also can occur with group A streptococcal infections at wound sites. The most common clinical presentation is **acute pharyngitis,** with a diffuse, erythematous **rash** of a sandpaper consistency developing on the second day of illness. The rash usually spares the face, palms, and soles and appears darker—so-called **Pastia's lines**—in skin folds of the axillae, groin, antecubital fossae, and knees. Other characteristic physical findings are a **strawberry tongue,** circumoral palor, and scattered petechiae. The skin rash fades with desquamation, usually after a week of illness. Eosinophilia may be present. Rarely, a severe form of scarlet fever associated with high fever and systemic toxicity, referred to as septic scarlet fever or toxic scarlet fever, may be accompanied by bacteremia, local wound infections, arthritis, and jaundice.

The diagnosis of scarlet fever is made by a positive throat culture for *S. pyogenes* and a compatible clinical syndrome. Treatment of scarlet fever is the same as for streptococcal pharyngitis. Penicillin remains the therapy of choice, although oral cephalosporins, erythromycin, and azithromycin are alternative choices. Penicillin is administered for 10 days to prevent acute rheumatic fever. The differential diagnosis of scarlet fever includes Kawasaki's disease, toxic shock syndrome, drug rash, and viral exanthems.

The present patient had a positive throat culture for group A streptococcus. This, coupled with her symptoms of fever, rash, pharyngitis, and strawberry tongue, confirmed the diagnosis of scarlet fever. She was treated with a 10-day course of penicillin V. Her rash gradually faded over the next 7 days and was followed by a superficial desquamation of her skin (see figure below).

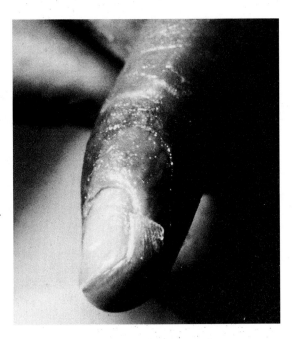

Clinical Pearls

1. The rash of scarlet fever has a sandpaper texture due to occlusion of sweat glands.
2. The rash of scarlet fever desquamates usually after a week of illness.
3. Eosinophilia may be seen in scarlet fever.

REFERENCES

1. Bartter T, Dascal A, Carroll K, et al: "Toxic strep syndrome"—A manifestation of group A streptococcal infection. Arch Intern Med 1988; 148:1421–1424.
2. Stevens DL, Tanner MH, Winship J, et al: Severe group A streptococcal infections associated with a toxic shock-like syndrome and scarlet fever toxin A. N Eng J Med 1989; 321:1–7.
3. Hoge CW, Schwartz B, Talkington DF, et al: The changing epidemiology of invasive group A streptococcal infections and the emergence of streptococcal toxic shock-like syndrome: A retrospective population-base study. JAMA 1993; 269:384–389.

PATIENT 38

A 30-year-old gardener with a nodular eruption on his arm

A 30-year-old man complains of painless nodules on his arm. He first noticed a lesion several weeks ago and was placed on cephalexin by his doctor. Lesions continued to appear despite antibiotic therapy. He denies fever, weight loss, and systemic complaints.

Physical Examination: Temperature 37°; pulse 70; respirations 14; blood pressure 130/70. General: well appearing, no distress. HEENT: normal. Cardiac: regular rhythm, no murmur. Chest: clear. Abdomen: soft, nontender, no organomegaly. Extremities: right arm has multiple, erythematous, papulonodular lesions, with a few ulcerating lesions along lymphatic channels (see figure).

Laboratory Findings: Hct 34%; WBC 10,000/μl with 75% neutrophils, 5% bands, 20% lymphocytes; hemoglobin 12 g/dl. Biopsy of lesion: pyogranulomas and cigar-shaped yeast forms.

Questions: What is the cause of this infection? How would you treat it?

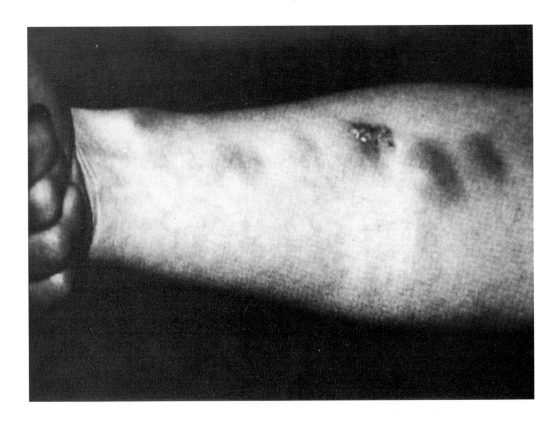

Diagnosis: Sporotrichosis

Discussion: This patient has nodular lymphangitis, which can develop after cutaneous inoculation of certain microorganisms into the body. *Sporothrix schenckii* was the first and most common organism to be associated with nodular lymphangitis, but many other organisms, including *Mycobacterium marinum, Nocardia* spp., *Mycobacterium kansasii, M. chelonei, M. avium-intracellulare, M. tuberculosis, Leishmania* spp., *Cryptococcus neoformans, Histoplasma capsulatum, Coccidioides immitis, Blastomyces dermatitis, Staphylococcus aureus, Francisella tularensis,* and cowpox virus, can produce similar disease.

S. schenckii and *M. marinum* are the most common causes of nodular lymphangitis. Sporotrichosis is a fungal infection caused by *S. schenckii* found in plants (especially roses) and soils in tropical and subtropical areas. Infection results from traumatic inoculation of the fungus into the skin. The most frequent clinical syndrome caused by sporotrichosis is cutaneous sporotrichosis, characterized by the appearance of papulonodular lesions often with lymphangitic spread. The incubation period is 1–2 weeks. Onset usually is indolent, with nodules developing over a period of weeks to months.

The lesions most often are painless, although mild tenderness may be present and ulceration can occur, and there are few systemic complaints. Extracutaneous sporotrichosis, which is rarely seen, can involve the bones, joints, lungs, eyes, and central nervous system in the normal or immunocompromised patient. Diagnosis is made by culturing the fungus from the lesions or by demonstrating the characteristic **cigar-shaped yeast forms** and **pyogranulomas** on biopsy. Lymphocutaneous sporotrichosis is treated with a saturated solution of potassium iodide (SSKI) or itraconazole. Amphotericin B should be used for extracutaneous sporotrichosis. Treatment must continue until all lesions are healed. Prolonged therapy (1–3 months) generally is required in the immunocompetent host.

M. marinum, a photochromogenic, acid-fast organism, causes infections in humans following exposure to fresh or salt water. Usually there is a preceding history of minor trauma or injury that occurred in a swimming pool or aquarium, followed by the appearance of mildly tender, papulonodular lesions 1–8 weeks later. The diagnosis is made by biopsy and culture of the lesion. Ethambutol, rifampin, trimethoprim-sulfamethoxazole (TMP-SMX), and minocycline have been used to treat this infection.

Nocardia species can cause cutaneous infection by direct inoculation. The typical presentation features a tender abscess or ulcerated papule, with nodular lesions appearing 2–4 weeks after trauma. Gram stain of purulent drainage shows thin, branching, gram-positive rods, and the definitive diagnosis is made by culturing *Nocardia*. Treatment is TMP-SMX, sulfadiazine, or minocycline.

The present patient was diagnosed with sporotrichosis based on the presence of papulonodular lesions, lymphangitic spread, and cigar-shaped yeast forms and pyogranulomas of *S. schenckii* on biopsy. He was treated with itraconazole for 3 months until all lesions were healed.

Clinical Pearls

1. The lesions of cutaneous sporotrichosis are painless.

2. Lymphocutaneous sporotrichosis must be distinguished from *Mycobacterium marinum* infection, nocardiosis, leishmaniasis, and tularemia.

3. Immunocompromised patients may develop multifocal, extracutaneous sporotrichosis.

REFERENCES

1. Caravalho J, Caldwell JB, Radford BL, Feldman AR: Feline-transmitted sporotrichosis in the southwestern United States. West J Med 1991; 154:462–465.
2. Sharkey-Mathis PK, Kauffman CA, Graybill JR, et al: Treatment of sporotrichosis with itraconazole. Rev Inf Dis 1991; 13:47–51.
3. Kostman JR, DiNubile MJ: Nodular lymphangitis: A distinctive but often unrecognized syndrome. Ann Intern Med 1993; 118:883–886.
4. Heller HM, Swartz NM: Nodular lymphangitis: Clinical features, differential diagnosis, and management. Curr Clin Topics Infect Dis 1994; 14:142–158.

PATIENT 39

A 50-year-old Puerto Rican woman with asthma, fever, and polymicrobial bacteremia

A 50-year-old woman born in Puerto Rico, with a long history of steroid-dependent asthma, comes to the emergency department with an acute asthmatic attack. Her last asthmatic attack was 3 weeks prior; she has been on prednisone since then. She complains of low-grade fever, a productive cough, and malaise, but denies abdominal pain, diarrhea, and night sweats. In the emergency department, her blood gas is pH 7.25, PCO_2 70 mmHg, PO_2 45 mmHg, and she is immediately intubated and transferred to the intensive care unit.

Physical Examination: Temperature 38.3°; pulse 140; respirations 30; blood pressure 150/90. General: obese; severe respiratory distress. HEENT: unremarkable. Cardiac: regular rate without murmur. Chest: diffuse rhonchi. Abdomen: soft, mild tenderness diffusely; positive bowel sounds. Extremities: no edema or rash.

Laboratory Findings: WBC 17,000/μl with 70% neutrophils, 20% bands, 10% lymphocytes. Chest radiograph: bilateral diffuse opacities. Blood cultures (two sets): gram-positive cocci and gram-negative rods. Bronchoscopy washings: filariform larvae (see figure).

Question: What clinical condition explains this patient's symptoms?

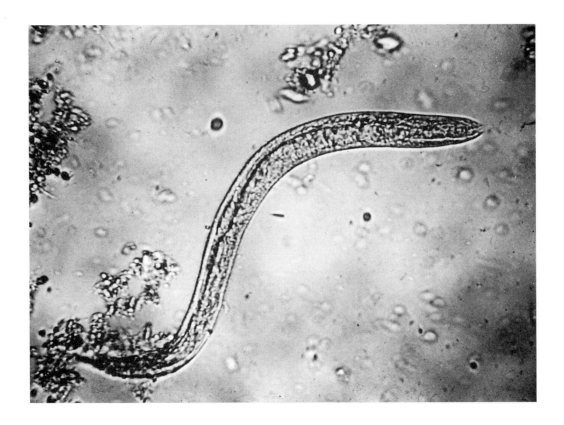

Diagnosis: Strongyloides hyperinfection syndrome

Discussion: Strongyloides stercoralis is a nematode that exists in the tropics and is especially common in Brazil, southeast Asia, and sub-Saharan Africa. The parasite is endemic in the southern United States, with an estimated prevalence of up to 4%. *S. stercoralis* can replicate in the human host and is able to persist for decades asymptomatically. However, in the immunocompromised host, overwhelming infection can occur with large numbers of larvae invading the lungs, gastrointestinal tract, and lymph nodes.

S. stercoralis has a complex life cycle. Humans are infected by **filariform larvae** found in contaminated soil. These larvae penetrate intact skin and pass by way of the bloodstream to the lungs, where they ascend the bronchial tree and then are swallowed, continuing into the small intestine. In the intestine, the larvae mature into adult females and penetrate the mucosa, where they deposit ova. In the normal host, rhabditiform larvae hatch, pass into the intestinal lumen, and are excreted with the feces. However, in immunosuppressed hosts, the rhabditiform larvae can transform into invasive filariform larvae in the intestine and penetrate the colonic mucosa, entering the blood stream to cause disseminated disease. This **autoinfection** results in hyperinfection syndrome, which frequently is accompanied by polymicrobial bactermia secondary to microperforations that occur in the gastrointestinal tract from larvae penetration.

Most patients with strongyloidiasis are **asymptomatic.** Some individuals develop a mild, itchy, urticarial rash, usually on the buttocks and wrists. Migrating larvae can produce a serpinginous, pruritic eruption called **larva currens,** which moves as the larvae migrate. Epigastric abdominal pain may be caused by the adult parasite burrowing into the small intestine mucosa and may be accompanied by mild weight loss, nausea, diarrhea, gastrointestinal bleeding, and mild colitis. In the normal host, pulmonary symptoms are unusual. Eosinophilia usually is present.

Immunosuppressed patients who develop disseminated strongyloidiasis may present with **gram-negative bacteremia or polymicrobial bacteremia, pneumonia, meningitis, colitis,** or **enteritis.** Eosinophilia typically is absent in overwhelming infection. In patients with pneumonia, bronchoscopy washings may demonstrate filariform larvae. Hyperinfection syndrome has been described in patients receiving long-term corticosteroids; with leukemia or lymphoma; and with acquired immunodeficiency syndrome.

Diagnosis of strongyloidiasis depends on demonstrating the characteristic larvae in feces or duodenal fluid in normal hosts, as well as in sputum and other tissues in immunocompromised patients. Multiple stool specimens should be sent in cases with a normal host because single stool examination is positive in only about 30% of patients.

The treatment of strongyloidiasis is **thiabendazole.** For treatment of the asymptomatic or normal host, a 2-day course of thiabendazole should be administered. Immunosuppressed patients with disseminated disease require a minimum 5–7 day course of therapy.

In the present patient, the diagnosis was made by visualizing filariform larvae in her bronchial washings. She was treated with a 7-day course of thiabendazole. After blood cultures grew enterococcus and *Escherichia coli,* ampicillin-sulbactam was prescribed for the bacteremia and pneumonia. The patient slowly improved over the next 2 weeks, and she was extubated and discharged home on the 21st hospital day.

Clinical Pearls

1. Polymicrobial bacteremia may occur in the hyperinfection syndrome of *Strongyloides.*

2. Eosinophilia is commonly present in the normal host with strongyloidiasis, but often is absent in the hyperinfection syndrome.

3. *S. stercoralis* can survive asymptomatically for many years in infected patients.

REFERENCES
1. Igra-Siegman Y, Kapila R, Sen P, et al: Syndrome of hyperinfection with *Strongyloides stercoralis.* Rev Infect Dis 1981; 3:397–407.
2. Genta RM: Global prevalence of strongyloidiasis: Critical review with epidemiologic insights into the prevention of disseminated disease. Rev Infect Dis 1989; 11:755.
3. Gompels MM: Disseminated strongyloidiasis in AIDS: Uncommon but important. AIDS 1991; 5:327.

PATIENT 40

A 30-year-old drug addict with fever, cough, and back pain

A 30-year-old intravenous drug user comes to the emergency department complaining of fever, cough, and severe back pain of 3-day duration. He also complains of a severe headache with neck stiffness. Past medical history is remarkable for heroin abuse. There are no known allergies. An HIV test was negative 3 months ago.

Physical Examination: Temperature 39.4°; pulse 120; respirations 30; blood pressure 110/70. General: moderately ill appearance. HEENT: conjunctival petechiae. Neck: nuchal rigidity. Cardiac: normal S_1S_2; grade III/VI holosystolic murmur, increases with inspiration. Chest: bilateral rhonchi. Abdomen: soft, nontender; pulsatile liver. Extremities: multiple, erythematous, purpuric lesions on fingers and toes.

Laboratory Findings: WBC 20,000/µl with 85% neutrophils, 10% bands, 5% lymphocytes; platelets 100,000/µl. Urinalysis: WBC 10/hpf, RBC 50/hpf, 2+ protein. Lumbar puncture: WBC 500/µl with 80% neutrophils, 20% lymphocytes; glucose 80 mg/dl; protein 150 mg/dl. CSF Gram stain: no organisms seen. Blood cultures (two sets): gram-positive cocci. Chest radiograph: multiple nodular opacities bilaterally (see figure).

Question: What diagnosis is most probable?

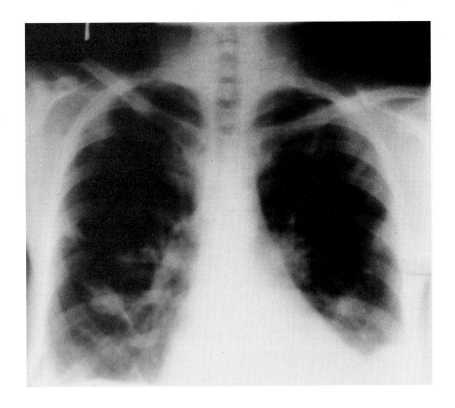

Diagnosis: Right-sided (tricuspid valve) *Staphylococcus aureus* endocarditis and septic emboli

Discussion: *S. aureus* is an important cause of both native valve and prosthetic valve endocarditis. *S. aureus* endocarditis in the **parenteral drug user** most commonly involves the tricuspid valve; in nonintravenous drug users, the mitral and aortic valves are more commonly involved. The tricuspid valve is involved alone or in combination with other valves in 50% of cases of infective endocarditis in drug addicts. The aortic valve is involved alone in 18%, aortic plus mitral in 12%, and only the mitral in 10%. The mortality and complication rates of left-sided *S. aureus* endocarditis approach 50%. Patients with right-sided *S. aureus* endocarditis have a much lower mortality rate and fewer complications from septic emboli.

The patient with tricuspid valve endocarditis typically presents with **pulmonary complaints** secondary to embolization of the lung. Patients may develop cough, pleuritic chest pain, pneumonia, hemoptysis from pulmonary infarct, or empyema. Up to 85% of intravenous drug users with right-sided *S. aureus* endocarditis have **abnormal chest films** showing septic pulmonary emboli.

Signs of tricuspid insufficiency are present in about 30%, with a pulsatile liver, gallop rhythm, large V waves, and holosystolic murmur that increases with inspiration. Embolic skin lesions, petechiae, Janeway's lesions, and splinter hemorrhages may be seen. **Neurologic manifestations** are commonly seen in *S. aureus* endocarditis. Cerebritis secondary to left-sided emboli or hematogenous spread of bacteria and aseptic or purulent meningitis may occur. The cerebrospinal fluid (CSF) is abnormal in about 15% of patients with endocarditis.

Endocarditis is characterized by a high-grade, persistent bacteremia. **Blood cultures are positive in close to 99%** of patients who have not recently received antibiotics. At least two sets of blood cultures should be drawn at separate sites.

A number of abnormal laboratory findings are typical. Anemia of chronic disease is seen in 90% of patients. Leukocytosis occurs in about 30%. The sedimentation rate is elevated in almost all patients. The urinalysis reveals proteinuria and microscopic hematuria in up to 60% of cases. Circulating immune complexes are present in most patients. The rheumatoid factor is positive in 50% of cases.

An electrocardiogram should be performed on admission because septal abscesses may cause various degrees of heart block. A transthoracic echocardiogram reveals vegetations in about 70% of patients, but transesophageal echocardiography has greater sensitivity and is the preferred procedure for visualizing prosthetic valves and complications such as valvular perforation or abscess.

The prognosis for right-sided endocarditis in the narcotic addict is good, with generally less than 5% mortality. The treatment of choice is **nafcillin** 2 g IV q4h combined with gentamicin for the first 5 days for synergy. The standard duration of therapy is 4 weeks, although a 2-week course may be curative. Several studies have shown that patients with right-sided endocarditis can be effectively treated with a 2-week course of nafcillin or oxacillin combined with gentamicin. An oral regimen of ciprofloxacin and rifampin for 4 weeks has been used to successfully treat ten intravenous drug users with right-sided *S. aureus* endocarditis; however the potential for quinolone resistance may limit this regimen.

The present patient was diagnosed with right-sided *S. aureus* endocarditis involving the tricuspid valve on the basis of the clinical findings (e.g., pulsatile liver, neck and back pain, embolic lesions, cough) and positive blood cultures. The patient's course was complicated by purulent meningitis, and the CSF culture also grew *S. aureus*. He was begun on high-dose nafcillin combined with gentamicin for the first 5 days for rapid clearing of bacteremia. Repeat blood cultures 3 days later were negative. An echocardiogram demonstrated a tricuspid vegetation. After initiation of antibiotics, the patient defervesced over 48 hours, and his headache and back pain resolved. Intravenous nafcillin was administered for a total of 4 weeks. Repeat blood cultures were sterile.

Clinical Pearls

1. Endocarditis in intravenous drug users involves the tricuspid valve in 50% of cases.

2. The most common symptoms of right-sided endocarditis are cough, dyspnea, and pleuritic chest pain.

3. The chest film in tricuspid valve endocarditis almost always is abnormal and frequently shows septic emboli.

4. Mortality is low in *S. aureus* right-sided endocarditis in IV drug users and high in *S. aureus* left-sided endocarditis in nonaddicts.

REFERENCES

1. Chambers HF: Short-course combination and oral therapies of *Staphylococcus aureus* endocarditis. Med Clin North Am 1993; 7:69–80.
2. Mortaora LA, Bayer AS: *Staphylococcus aureus* bacteremia and endocarditis: New diagnostic and therapeutic concepts. Infect Dis Clin North 1993; 7:53–68.
3. Wilson WR, Karchmer MD, Dajani AS, et al: Antibiotic treatment of adults with infective endocarditis due to streptococci, enterococci, staphylococci, and HACEK microorganisms. JAMA 1995; 274:1706–1713.
4. Cunha BA, Gill MV, Lazar JM: Acute infective endocarditis. Infect Dis Clin North Am 1996; 10:811–834.

PATIENT 41

A 50-year-old diabetic man with a foot ulcer

A 50-year-old man with a history of diabetes mellitus complains of a nonhealing ulcer on the plantar surface of his left foot. He first noted the ulcer about 2 weeks prior to his visit, after discovering a purulent discharge staining his sock. In addition, he has experienced some swelling and redness of the dorsum of his foot. A low-grade fever has been present for 2–3 days. He denies any pain, and cannot recall any specific trauma to the area. After noting the ulcer, he had visited a podiatrist who prescribed a "salve," but the patient did not keep his follow-up appointment. His past medical history is significant for diabetes mellitus of 15-year duration, with known complications of peripheral neuropathy, retinopathy, and chronic renal insufficiency. He is currently taking glyburide and captopril for hypertension. He denies any drug allergies.

Physical Examination: Temperature 37.8°; pulse 84; respirations 14; blood pressure 160/95. HEENT: extensive retinal scarring due to prior laser photocoagulation. Cardiac: normal. Abdomen: unremarkable. Extremities: hairless below knees, multiple ecchymoses in various stages of resolution, dorsalis pedis and posterior tibial pulses diminished bilaterally, 2+ right pedal edema with overlying erythema; well-circumscribed, punched-out ulcer approximately 2½ inches in diameter on plantar surface of left foot over area of second metatarsal head, with devitalized tissue and purulent discharge.

Laboratory Findings: WBC 15,300/μl with 88% neutrophils, 2% bands, 9% lymphocytes, 1% monocytes. BUN 24 mg/dl, creatinine 2.3 mg/dl. ESR 98 mm/hr. Culture of foot ulcer: *Staphylococcus aureus, S. epidermidis, Escherichia coli,* and *Enterococcus.* Radiograph of left foot: see figure.

Question: What is your diagnosis?

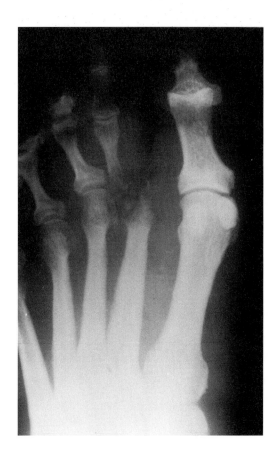

Diagnosis: Diabetic foot ulcer with chronic osteomyelitis

Discussion: Diabetic foot infections, when limited to the skin or superficial soft tissues, are caused by the same pathogens as in nondiabetics. These pathogens include *S. aureus*, streptococci, *E. coli* and other enteric gram-negative bacilli, and enterococci. In the diabetic patient with deep, penetrating infections, a variety of anaerobic pathogens such as *Peptostreptococcus, Peptococcus,* fusobacteria, and *Bacteroides* spp. must also be considered.

Diabetics presenting with deep, penetrating ulcers or chronic, draining sinus tracts of the foot almost always have an underlying chronic osteomyelitis. Even carefully taken cultures of the ulcer or sinus tract represent surface colonization and should not be equated with the underlying pathologic process or the presumed pathogenic organism. Only **bone biopsy cultures** are diagnostic and can be relied upon to select or change antibiotic therapy. Therefore, bone biopsy always should be performed. Prolonged empiric therapy should be avoided. **Extensive surgical debridement,** in addition to appropriate antimicrobial therapy, invariably is required for cure of chronic osteomyelitis. Inadequate debridement, in the hopes of preserving cosmesis, results in persistent or worsening infection despite prolonged antibiotics.

Initial empiric antibiotic therapy should consist of a broad-spectrum agent that has activity against the organisms mentioned above. Monotherapy with a third-generation cephalosporin (e.g., cefotaxime, ceftizoxime, cefoperazone) or a penicillin-β-lactamase inhibitor combination (e.g., ampicillin/sulbactam, piperacillin/tazobactam, ticarcillin/clavulanate) provides appropriate coverage. In the penicillin-allergic patient, clindamycin in combination with an aminoglycoside, quinolone, or aztreonam is recommended. Generally, monotherapy with an older quinolone should not be relied upon because of potential development of resistance, especially in staphylococci. Trovafloxacin, a broad-spectrum quinolone, is an exception to this rule. Although a small percentage of diabetic foot infections are caused by *Pseudomonas aeruginosa*, empiric coverage for this organism is not warranted. *P. aeruginosa* should be suspected, however, in cases following puncture wounds through a sneaker, and double *Pseudomonas* coverage should be initiated pending culture in this situation.

The present patient's foot ulcer—of prolonged duration—in combination with a **markedly elevated ESR** is suspicious for an underlying osteomyelitis. The destructive bony changes on radiograph confirm the diagnosis. If the radiograph had been nondiagnostic, a technetium bone scan would have been indicated. The patient underwent a ray amputation of the second phalanx and distal metatarsal bone. While an inpatient, he was given a week of IV ampicillin/sulbactam, which subsequently was changed to an oral combination of clindamycin and ofloxacin for an additional 3 weeks outpatient.

Clinical Pearls

1. In a diabetic with a nonhealing foot ulcer, an elevated ESR is suspicious for underlying osteomyelitis.

2. Superficial cultures rarely are helpful in establishing the pathogenic organism in osteomyelitis complicating a diabetic foot ulcer. A bone biopsy culture should be performed to direct antimicrobial therapy.

3. Extensive surgical debridement *always* is required for cure in cases of chronic osteomyelitis.

4. Empiric anti-*Pseudomonas* therapy is only necessary for patients who have experienced puncture wounds through a sneaker.

REFERENCES
1. Caputo GM, Cavanagh PR, Ulbrecht JS, et al: Diabetic foot infections. N Engl J Med 1994; 331:854–860.
2. Cunha BA: Diabetic foot infections. Infect Dis Pract 1994; 18:39.
3. Gibbens GW, Havershaw GM: Diabetic foot infections. Infect Dis Clin North Am 1995; 9:131–142.

PATIENT 42

A 60-year-old man with chronic lung disease and bilateral lower lobe opacities

A 60-year-old man with a history of chronic obstructive pulmonary disease (COPD) presents with complaints of cough and increasing dyspnea over the past 4 days. The cough initially was nonproductive, but during the previous 24 hours it has become mucopurulent, with copious yellow-green sputum production. Last night the patient developed a fever, up to 38.8°C, and chills. He denies pleuritic pain and hemoptysis. His past medical history is significant for nonsteroid-dependent COPD of 10-year duration. He continues to smoke one pack of cigarettes per day. His only current medication is ipratropium bromide inhaler (2 puffs qid). He has no drug allergies.

Physical Examination: Temperature 38.4°; pulse 115; respirations 24; blood pressure 140/86. Chest: lung bases dull to percussion, bibasilar rales and scattered wheezes in both lungs.

Laboratory Findings: Hct 44%; WBC 14,800/μl with 82% neutrophils, 7% bands, 11% lymphocytes. Electrolytes, BUN, creatinine: normal. Arterial blood gas: pH 7.42, PCO_2 32 mmHg, PO_2 58 mmHg. Sputum Gram stain: see figure (left). Chest radiograph: see figure (right).

Questions: What is the likely etiology of this patient's pneumonia? What antibiotics would you begin, empirically?

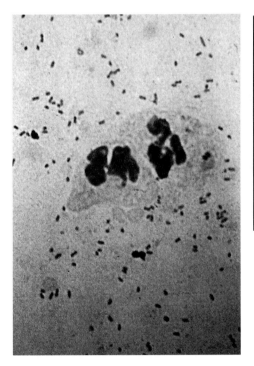

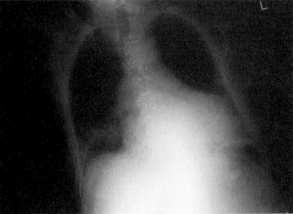

Diagnosis: *Hemophilus influenzae* pneumonia

Discussion: *H. influenzae* is a pleomorphic, gram-negative coccobacillus that is a major human pathogen, causing many cases of acute otitis media, sinusitis in children, and both upper and lower respiratory tract infections in adults. There are six capsular serotypes of *H. influenzae,* of which serotype b (Hib) is the primary human pathogen. The incidence of Hib-related disease, most notably bacterial meningitis in infants and toddlers, has declined significantly since the introduction of an effective vaccine in 1991. Unencapsulated *H. influenzae,* also termed nontypable *H. influenzae* (NTHi), is implicated in the majority of *H. influenzae*-associated respiratory infections. It causes disease primarily by damaging the epithelial cells in the respiratory mucosa.

H. influenzae can colonize the respiratory tracts of healthy children and adults, but the rates of colonization are much greater in persons with COPD (50–60%). Colonization can last for weeks to months. In patients with COPD, the same isolate can be found in respiratory secretions, even after successful treatment with antibiotics to which the organism is sensitive. The majority of patients with *H. influenzae* pneumonia or acute tracheobronchitis have underlying COPD. Other risk factors include pregnancy, human immunodeficiency virus infection, and malignancy.

The clinical features of pneumonia due to *H. influenzae* are essentially indistinguishable from those of other bacterial pneumonias. Fever, cough, and purulent sputum production usually are present. Radiographic appearance is nonspecific, but **lower lobe involvement** is typical. Gram stain of the sputum can be diagnostic, since the organism usually is profuse in respiratory secretions of patients without prior antibiotic therapy. Blood cultures are positive in about 15% of cases due to NTHi. Hib, when responsible for infection, is more likely to invade the bloodstream.

β-lactamase-mediated resistance is a feature of 20–50% of *H. influenzae* isolates and is approximately twice as common in Hib than in NTHi strains. Infections due to ampicillin-resistant strains can be effectively managed with ampicillin/β-lactamase inhibitors, TMP/SMX, a second- or third-generation cephalosporin, or a quinolone. In addition, NTHi strains remain almost uniformly sensitive to the second-generation tetracyclines, doxycycline and minocycline. Doxycycline's effectiveness against these nontypable strains of *H. influenzae,* as well as against *Streptococcus pneumoniae* and *Moraxella catarrhalis,* make it a good alternative agent in the treatment of community-acquired pneumonia, even in patients with COPD.

The present patient demonstrated lower lobe involvement on chest radiograph, and sputum Gram stain revealed *H. influenzae* colonization. He was admitted to the hospital and started empirically on ceftriaxone, 1 g (IV) q24 hours, and supplemental oxygen therapy. He defervesced over the subsequent 48 hours, and the WBC returned to normal. After 3 days of intravenous antibiotics, he was switched to amoxicillin/clavulanate, 875 mg bid, and completed therapy as an outpatient.

Clinical Pearls

1. *H. influenzae* can colonize the upper respiratory tract for weeks to months. Rates of colonization approach 60% in persons with underlying COPD.

2. Nontypable strains account for about 80% of the upper and lower respiratory tract infections caused by *H. influenzae.*

3. β-lactamase production can be found in up to 50% of ampicillin-resistant strains of *H. influenzae.* Alternative therapies include ampicillin/β-lactamase inhibitor combinations, most cephalosporins, trimethoprim/sulfamethoxazole, a quinolone, doxycycline, or a newer macrolide/azalide antibiotic.

REFERENCES
1. Takala AK, Eskola J, van Alphen L: Spectrum of invasive *Haemophilus influenzae* type b disease in adults. Arch Intern Med 1990; 150:2573–2576.
2. Farley MM, Stephens DS, Brachman PS, et al: Invasive *H. influenzae* disease in adults: A prospective population based surveillance. Ann Intern Med 1992; 116:806–812.
3. Kostman JR, Sherry BL, Fligner CL, et al: Invasive *Haemophilus influenzae* in older children and adults in Seattle. Clin Infect Dis 1993; 17:389–396.

PATIENT 43

A 60-year-old man with fever and right-sided pleural effusion

A 60-year-old man presents with a 2-day history of fever, shaking chills, nausea, and right-sided pleuritic chest pain. He denies dyspnea and cough. He has a history of diet-controlled diabetes mellitus and is status post cholecystectomy (surgery 2 months previously).

Physical Examination: Temperature 39.5°; pulse 120; respirations 18. General: ill-appearing. HEENT: unremarkable. Chest: decreased breath sounds and dullness to percussion at right base, no rales or rhonchi. Cardiac: no murmur. Abdomen: soft; mild right upper quadrant tenderness; slight hepatomegaly (14 cm in midclavicular line); no splenomegaly. Skin: no rash. Lymph nodes: normal. Extremities: no calf tenderness noted.

Laboratory Examination: Hct 36%; WBC 15,200/μl with 72% neutrophils, 19% bands, 3% lymphocytes, 6% monocytes. Electrolytes, BUN, creatinine: normal. ESR 82 mm/hr, aspartate aminotransferase 82 IU/L, alanine aminotransferase 55 IU/L. Alkaline phosphatase 122 IU/L. Chest radiograph: small right pleural effusion that layers freely on decubitus positioning. Blood cultures: gram-negative rods, identification pending. Abdominal CT scan: see figure.

Question: What diagnosis might explain this patient's symptoms and radiologic abnormalities?

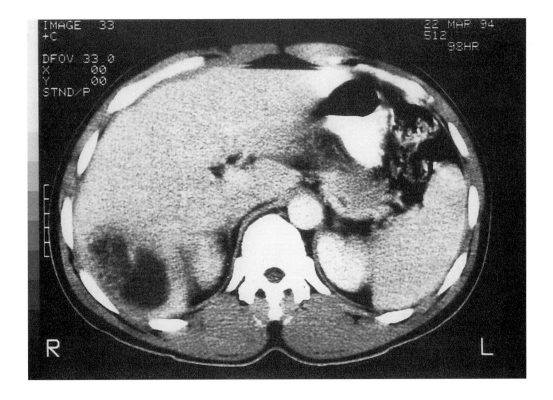

Diagnosis: Pyogenic liver abscess with *Escherichia coli* bacteremia

Discussion: Pyogenic liver abscess is a rare, but potentially life-threatening, infection. In the post-antibiotic era, pyogenic liver abscesses occur most frequently in middle-aged and elderly patients as a complication of underlying **biliary tract disease.** As many as 15–20% of cases are considered cryptogenic, however. Up to 70% of abscesses are localized to the **right hepatic lobe,** with the majority of these being solitary lesions. Multiple abscesses, when they occur, often are found in patients with severe underlying tract disease states.

Among the known causes of pyogenic liver abscess, biliary tract disease is the most common, accounting for about one-third of cases. This disease may be of benign or malignant origin, arising from conditions such as cholelithiasis, choledocholithiasis, sclerosing cholangitis, cholangiocarcinoma, and pancreatic carcinoma. Hematogenous infection may occur via the hepatic artery or, more commonly, via the portal circulation from diverticulitis, appendicitis, pancreatic and splenic infections, and other intra-abdominal infections. Direct extension from a contiguous site can take place, as in penetrating tumors and duodenal ulcers. Secondary infection of hepatic cysts, tumors, metastatic lesions, and granulomas may occur, and blunt or penetrating trauma also may predispose to localized infection.

The most frequent presenting symptoms are fever, malaise, anorexia, abdominal pain, rigors, nausea, and vomiting. Additional symptoms include weight loss, night sweats, diarrhea, dyspnea, cough, and pleurisy. **Hepatomegaly** is present in more than 50% of patients, with right upper quadrant tenderness, jaundice, abdominal distension, variable elevations of serum transaminases and alkaline phosphatase, mild anemia, and an elevated ESR. Chest radiographs are abnormal in approximately 50% of patients, revealing a right pleural effusion, right basilar atelectasis, or elevated hemidiaphragm.

Imaging techniques used in the diagnosis of hepatic abscess include technetium-99 radionuclide scanning, ultrasonography, and **CT scanning**. CT is generally considered the most sensitive method for detecting hepatic abscesses, with a sensitivity of 88–97% when intravenous contrast is utilized.

The bacteriology of hepatic abscess has changed drastically over the past two decades, mostly due to improved laboratory culturing techniques. **Polymicrobial infection** is present in up to 64% of cases and is especially common in solitary abscess cultures. Major bacterial isolates include *E. coli* (37%), *Staphylococcus aureus* (23%), *Streptococcus* sp. (17%), *Proteus* sp. (13%), and *Klebsiella* or *Enterobacter* sp. (12%). Anaerobes are present in approximately 50% of liver abscesses. So-called sterile abscesses probably reflect a lack of adequate anaerobic culture techniques.

Small liver abscesses may be treated with prolonged courses of antibiotics, often requiring 4–6 weeks of therapy. Appropriate therapy covers those organisms likely involved, including streptococci, enteric gram-negative rods, and anaerobes. In the setting of trauma or surgery, antistaphylococcal antibiotics are required. Large abscess cavities should be drained surgically or, when feasible, via CT-guided percutaneous aspiration. Antimicrobial therapy should be continued until complete shrinkage of the abscess is documented on follow-up CT scans.

The present patient was started initially on IV ampicillin/sulbactam. Because of his abnormal liver enzymes and right upper quadrant tenderness, a CT scan of the abdomen was obtained. This image revealed a large, solitary abscess in the right lobe of the liver. A percutaneous aspirate yielded approximately 30 cc of purulent material, which grew *E. coli* on culture. A pigtail stent was left in place until resolution of the abscess cavity was documented on follow-up CT. After 7 days, the antibiotics were changed to a combination of oral ciprofloxacin and metronidazole for a 3-week course. The patient was discharged on day 8, with no further complications.

Clinical Pearls

1. When faced with a patient demonstrating fever and pleural effusion in the absence of a pneumonic process, always consider a subdiaphragmatic abscess.

2. Underlying biliary tract disease is the most common cause of pyogenic liver abscesses, but up to 20% are considered cryptogenic.

3. Surgical or percutaneous drainage—for both diagnostic and therapeutic purposes—and broad-spectrum antimicrobial therapy are essential for cure of moderate-to-large liver abscesses.

4. Enteric gram-negative rods, enterococci, microaerophilic streptococci, *S. aureus,* and anaerobes are the most commonly isolated organisms.

REFERENCES

1. McDonald AP, Howare RJ: Pyogenic liver abscess. World J Surg 1980; 4:369–380.
2. McDonald MI, Corey GR, Gallis HA, Durack DT: Single and multiple pyogenic liver abscesses: Natural history, diagnosis, and treatment, with emphasis on percutaneous drainage. Medicine 1984; 63:291–302.
3. Branum GD, Tyson GS, Branum MA, Meyers WC: Hepatic abscess: Changes in etiology, diagnosis, and management. Ann Surg 1990; 212:655–662.

PATIENT 44

A 32-year-old man with abdominal cramps, flatulence, and diarrhea

A 32-year-old man presents with complaints of persistent diarrhea associated with severe abdominal cramping and flatulence of 4-day duration. He has noted six to seven watery bowel movements per day, but denies the presence of mucus or blood. During the first day of illness, he was nauseous and vomited twice. Two weeks ago he returned from a camping trip in the Colorado mountains, where he was bitten by mosquitoes and ticks, ate wild berries, and drank from a cold mountain stream. He has not noticed any fever or chills. Past medical history is unremarkable.

Physical Examination. Temperature 36.7°; pulse 95; respirations 16; blood pressure 110/70. HEENT: mucous membranes somewhat dry. Chest, cardiac, extremities: normal; no rash or lymphadenopathy. Abdomen: mildly protuberant; tympanitic with slightly increased bowel sounds; mild, diffuse tenderness on deep palpation; no organomegaly. Rectal: no stool in rectal vault.

Laboratory Examination: Hct 44%; WBC 9600/μl with 82% neutrophils, 16% lymphocytes, 2% monocytes; platelets 202,000/μl. Na^+ 142 mEq/L, K^+ 3.2 mEq/L, Cl^- 112 mEq/L, HCO_3^- 19 mEq/L. Liver function tests: unremarkable. Stool: fecal leukocyte stain negative.

Question: What is the likely diagnosis?

Diagnosis: Giardiasis

Discussion: Giardiasis, caused by the protozoa *Giardia lamblia,* is one of the most common parasitic diseases worldwide, causing endemic and epidemic intestinal disease and diarrhea. Infection occurs after ingestion of the cyst form of the organism, which remains in the proximal small bowel and releases the trophozoite forms. Only a small number of cysts are required for effective transmission to humans. **Waterborne transmission** accounts for most episodic infections, with the cysts remaining viable for long periods in cold water and resisting routine chlorination methods. In the United States, *Giardia* remains the most frequent cause of waterborne gastroenteritis outbreaks.

Clinically, giardiasis ranges from asymptomatic carriage to severe diarrheal illness with malabsorption. Acute giardiasis develops following a 1–3 week incubation period. Diarrhea, bloating, abdominal cramps, belching, flatus, nausea, and vomiting are prominent early symptoms. Diarrhea often subsides after about 1 week, but chronic giardiasis may occur, with prolonged or recurrent episodes of symptoms. A small number of infected patients develop subsequent lactose intolerance or malabsorption. Patients with hypogammaglobulinemia commonly suffer from prolonged, severe infections that respond poorly to treatment regimens.

Physical examination usually is not helpful in diagnosing giardiasis. Exposure to fresh water sources in the environment or contact with infected individuals in an institutional setting, such as a day care center, often is illicited in the clinical history. The presence of fever and blood or mucus in the stool should prompt the consideration of alternative diagnoses. The diagnosis is made by finding cysts or trophozoites in the feces or small intestine. **Multiple stool examinations, duodenal aspirates, or small bowel biopsy may be required.** Commercial tests (immunofluorescent or enzyme-linked immunosorbent assays) for *Giardia* antigens in the stool are now available.

Metronidazole, 250 mg tid for 5 days, is the recommended therapy for the treatment of giardiasis. Quinacrine is equally effective. Cure rates exceed 80%. Treatment failures often can be successfully managed with a longer course of the initial drug. Those patients with persistent or recurrent infection should be evaluated for repeated exposure from close contacts or environmental sources and for the presence of hypogammaglobulinemia.

The present patient was noted to have *Giardia lamblia* trophozoites on trichrome stain of a fresh stool sample. He was treated with a standard course of metronidazole and recovered uneventfully.

Clinical Pearls

1. The protozoa *Giardia lamblia* is the most common cause of waterborne outbreaks of diarrheal illness in the United States.

2. In symptomatic giardiasis, belching, bloating, flatus, and abdominal cramping are often the most prominent symptoms.

3. Lactose intolerance or malabsorption may complicate the course of giardiasis in some patients, and may persist after elimination of the organism.

4. Fever and blood or mucus in the stool is *not* a feature of *Giardia* infection.

5. Although diagnosis often is made on examination of fresh stool, duodenal aspirates or biopsy may be required.

6. Hypogammaglobulinemia predisposes an individual to severe or relapsing infection and predicts a risk for treatment failure.

REFERENCES
1. Wolfe MS: Giardiasis. Clin Microbiol Rev 1992; 5:92–100.
2. Hill DR: Giardiasis: Issues in diagnosis and management. Infect Dis Clin North Am 1993; 7:503–525.

PATIENT 45

A 42-year-old woman with erythema nodosum, abdominal pain, and diarrhea

A 42-year-old woman is admitted to the surgical service in your hospital for possible appendicitis. Three days prior to admission she experienced sudden onset of watery diarrhea associated with crampy abdominal pain and fever to 38.8°C. She limited herself to a liquid diet, but noted persistent fever and steadily increasing pain that localized to the right lower quadrant over the subsequent 2 days. This morning she observed two painful red areas, unrelated to trauma, on her right shin. She denies nausea, vomiting, tenesmus, and blood in the stool. She lives alone, has no pets, denies recent travel, and has not ingested undercooked meats, shellfish, or any type of "fast food" in the previous week. Past medical history is unremarkable.

The patient is being prepped for a laparoscopic appendectomy.

Physical Examination: Temperature 38.5°; pulse 120; respirations 18; blood pressure 110/60. General: acutely ill, mildly dehydrated. Chest: normal. Cardiac: normal. Abdomen: bowel sounds slightly hyperactive; voluntary guarding; tenderness of right lower quadrant, but no rebound tenderness. Rectum: no stool in vault. Extremities: two tender, erythematous nodules on right anterior tibia.

Laboratory Findings: Hct 35%; WBC 16, 400/µl with 82% neutrophils, 3% bands, 14% lymphocytes, 1% monocytes. Serum electrolytes: normal. BUN 45 mg/dl, creatinine 1.1 mg/dl. Liver function tests and urinalysis: normal. Serum pregnancy test: negative. Radiographs (flat and upright of abdomen): nonspecific gas pattern in bowel, no evidence of free air.

Question: What is the most likely clinical diagnosis?

Diagnosis: Mesenteric adenitis (pseudoappendicitis) due to *Yersinia enterocolitica*

Discussion: *Y. enterocolitica* is a gram-negative, nonlactose-fermenting, urease-positive bacilli. Although a relatively uncommon cause of infectious diarrhea in the United States, *Y. enterocolitica* is implicated in 1–3% of cases of bacterial enteritis worldwide, most frequently in northern Europe. The bacteria's portal of entry is the oropharynx or gastrointestinal tract, with outbreaks reported from both food and water sources. Many domestic animals serve as reservoirs for the organism, and animal-to-person or person-to-person transmission is common.

Enterocolitis is the most common manifestation of disease, characterized by fever, diarrhea, and abdominal pain lasting 1–3 weeks. Blood or mucus in the stool is rare, occurring usually in neonates and young children. When blood or fecal leukocytes are present, an alternative pathogen should be considered. The syndrome of mesenteric adenitis is characterized by **fever, leukocytosis,** and **right lower quadrant pain** that may be clinically indistinguishable from appendicitis (thus the term "pseudoappendicitis"). This syndrome typically occurs in older children and young adults.

In Scandinavia, a reactive polyarthritis occurs in 10–30% of adult patients with mesenteric adenitis, usually beginning several days to a month after the onset of diarrhea. The HLA-B27 histocompatibility antigen is present in about 65% of these patients. **Erythema nodosum** can be associated with adult *Yersinia* infections, especially in women over age 40. Erythema nodosum is present in up to 30% of Scandinavian cases. Lesions typically appear on the legs and trunk 2–20 days after the onset of diarrhea and abdominal pain and resolve spontaneously within a month.

Y. enterocolitica septicemia is a less frequent manifestation of disease. It is reported most often in patients with underlying disease states such as diabetes mellitus, cirrhosis, malignancy, or severe anemia. Patients with iron overload (e.g., hemochromatosis) are particularly prone to bacteremia. Desferrioxamine, an iron chelator used in treating these patients, enhances the growth of *Y. enterocolitica.*

Although there are many conditions that associate with erythema nodosum (see table at right) or mimic appendicitis (see table on next page), very few conditions do both. Those of infectious etiology include *Y. enterocolitica, Campylobacter jejuni,* and *Salmonella* gastroenteritis. Of these, only *Y. enterocolitica* is implicated frequently enough to warrant its consideration as the likely pathogen. Of the noninfectious conditions, only Crohn's disease is associated with both pseudoappendicitis and erythema nodosum.

Conditions Associated with Erythema Nodosum

Infections	Inflammatory/Autoimmune
Streptococcal infections (usually tonsillo pharyngitis)`	Inflammatory bowel disease
	Ulcerative colitis
	Crohn's disease
Tuberculosis	Systemic lupus
Mycoses	erythematosus
Coccidioidomycosis	Drugs
	Sulfonamides and other
Blastomycosis	sulfa-class drugs
Histoplasmosis	Halides (bromides,
Trichophyton spp.	iodides)
superficial	Oral contraceptives
infections	Barbiturates
Viruses	Sarcoidosis
Hepatitis B	Malignancy
EBV mononucleosis	Lymphoma
	Hodgkin's disease
Chlamydia	Non-Hodgkin's
Lymphogranuloma venereum	lymphoma
	Leukemia
Psittacosis	
Rickettsia	
Other bacteria	
Yersinia infections (arthritis, gastroenteritis)	
Campylobacter jejuni	
Salmonella species (gastroenteritis)	
Cat scratch disease	
Tularemia	

EBV = Epstein-Barr virus

Obtaining positive cultures of *Y. enterocolitica* from stool, blood, or mesenteric lymph nodes confirms the diagnosis. When *Y. enterocolitica* is strongly suspected, the microbiology laboratory should be notified, since the use of selective media and other techniques can increase the yield of positive cultures. Hemagglutination titers can be diagnostic, but are less timely, and they can cross react with species of *Brucella, Salmonella* spp., and *Vibrio cholerae.*

In most cases, the enteritis associated with *Y. enterocolitica* is self-limited. Treatment is advocated in those patients with severe disease or bacteremia and may shorten the length of illness and duration of shedding of the organism. A third-generation cephalosporin or an aminoglycoside is considered the treatment of choice. A fluoroquinolone is an effective alternative agent.

The present patient's fever and right lower quadrant pain suggested appendicitis, but the diarrhea warranted further investigation. A CT examination of the abdomen revealed enlarged mesenteric lymph nodes and inflammation of the terminal ileum; the appendix was unremarkable. Stool cultures were positive for *Y. enterocolitica,* and the lesions were identified as erythema nodosum associated with *Y. enterocolitica* infection. Therapy with intravenous cefotaxime and fluids was instituted. The patient's diarrhea improved, and the erythema nodosum gradually faded over the subsequent 10 days.

The Differential Diagnosis of Pseudoappendicitis

Noninfectious Causes	Infectious Causes	
Crohn's disease	Measles (pre-eruptive)	Typhlitis
Hypergammaglobulinemia	*Yersinia enterocolitica*	Diverticulitis
IgD syndrome	*Campylobacter jejuni*	Salpingitis
Diabetic ketoacidosis	*Plesiomonas* shigelloides	Right-sided tubo-ovarian
Luetic crisis	*Salmonella heidelberg*	abscess
Porphyria (acute)	*Vibrio hollisae*	Amoeboma
Acute pancreatitis	Typhoid fever	Actinomycosis
Acute cholecystitis	Typhoidal tularemia	Rocky Mountain spotted
(low-lying gallbladder)	Typhoidal EBV	fever
Vasculitis	mononucleosis	Bubonic plague
Small bowel hematoma	Scarlet fever (right	Legionnaires' disease
	rectus syndrome)	Parvovirus B19

EBV = Epstein Barr virus

Clinical Pearls

1. Although accounting for only 1–3% of cases of bacterial enteritis worldwide, *Y. enterocolitica* is the predominant organism associated with the syndrome of mesenteric adenitis ("pseudoappendicitis").

2. Reactive polyarthritis complicates up to 30% of adult cases in Scandinavia. The presence of the HLA-B27 antigen is a predisposing factor.

3. Up to 30% of patients with *Y. enterocolitica* infection also have erythema nodosum, and the association is most common in women over age 40.

4. Iron overload states predispose to severe *Y. enterocolitica* infection. Treatment with iron-chelating agents increases this risk.

REFERENCES

1. Cover TL, Aber RC: *Yersinia enterocolitica*. N Engl J Med 1989; 321:16–24.
2. Bisset J, Powers LC, Abbot SL, et al: Epidemiologic investigations of *Yersinia enterocolitica* and related species: Sources, frequency, and serogroup distribution. J Clin Microbiol 1990; 28:910–912.
3. Van Noyen R, Selderslaghs R, Bekaert J, et al: Causative role of *Yersinia* and other enteric pathogens in the appendicular syndrome. Eur J Clin Microbiol Infect Dis 1991; 10:735–741.

PATIENT 46

A 65-year-old man with fever, headache, and right hemiparesis

A 65-year-old man is admitted to the hospital with dysarthria and right hemiparesis that have progressed over a 12-hour period. Prior to the onset of weakness, he complained of a left frontotemporal headache lasting several days, relating it to his "sinus problems." Since the onset of the current symptoms, he has experienced nausea and vomited twice. He denies fever, chills, neck stiffness, photophobia, and recent trauma. He has had multiple transient ischemic attacks in the past, and he underwent a left carotid endarterectomy 3 years previously.

The remainder of the past medical history is significant for chronic stable angina pectoris, mild hypertension, and diet-controlled diabetes mellitus. Current medications include amoxicillin/clavulanate and terfenadine (started 5 days ago) for recurrent sinusitis, isosorbide dinitrate, and nitroglycerine tablets. There is no history of drug allergy.

Physical Examination: Temperature 37.9°; pulse 115; respirations 18; blood pressure 134/85. General: lethargic, mildly confused. HEENT: tympanic membranes and oropharynx normal, no sinus tenderness, transillumination of sinuses equivocal. Neck: supple, well-healed endarterectomy scar, mild bruit over right carotid artery. Chest: lungs clear. Cardiac and abdomen: unremarkable. Extremities: 1+ pedal edema bilaterally. Neurologic: mild left facial weakness and notable dysarthria; sensory intact, but motor strength of right upper and lower extremities diminished (grade 2/5); slight hyperreflexia on right side.

Laboratory Findings: Hct 33%; WBC 9800/μl with 75% neutrophils, 20% lymphocytes, 4% monocytes, 1% eosinophils. Na$^+$ 130 mEq/L, K$^+$ 4.2 mEq/L, Cl$^-$ 96 mEq/L, HCO$_3^-$ 24 mEq/L. BUN 24 mg/dl, creatinine 1.0 mg/dl. Urinalysis: normal. ESR 54 mm/hr.

Questions: What is the leading diagnosis? What is the next step in the workup of this patient?

Answers: Brain abscess secondary to paranasal sinusitis. A computed tomography scan of the head should be performed immediately.

Discussion: Brain abscess is a rare condition, but should always be suspected in patients with **fever, headache, and focal neurologic deficit.** A brain abscess can arise from intracranial extension of infection from a contiguous site, after hematogenous spread from a distant focus, or secondary to direct trauma or surgery. The etiology in up to 20% of patients remains cryptogenic. Contiguous infections that predispose to abscess formation include paranasal sinusitis, otitis media and mastoiditis, and dental infections (usually following molar extractions). Most otogenic abscesses are located in the temporal lobe or cerebellum, while sinus disease usually is associated with a frontal lobe abscess. Extension from sphenoid sinusitis also may affect the temporal lobe or sella turcica. **Sinusitis** remains the major predisposing condition leading to subdural empyema.

Hematogenous brain abscesses typically are multiple and multiloculated. Predisposing conditions include chronic pyogenic lung diseases, such as bronchiectasis or empyema, infective endocarditis, congenital heart disease, and pulmonary arteriovenous malformations. These conditions presumably allow septic microemboli direct access to the cerebral circulation.

Pyogenic brain abscesses are polymicrobial in up to 60% of cases. Various streptococci commonly are found, often in combination with gram-negative enteric bacilli and anaerobes, including *Bacteroides fragilis. Staphylococcus aureus,* in pure culture, causes the majority of complications associated with trauma or neurosurgical procedures. Interestingly, those organisms responsible for most cases of bacterial meningitis (*Streptococcus pneumoniae, Hemophilus influenzae*) rarely cause brain abscesses.

Clinically, the classic triad of fever, headache, and focal neurologic deficit occurs in less than 50%. Most patients have a moderate-to-severe **headache,** and fever occurs in about half. Changes in mental status, ranging from mild drowsiness to coma, are common. The preoperative mental status of the patient directly correlates with overall mortality. Nausea and vomiting, due to increased intracranial pressure, is found in about 50% of cases, while papilledema occurs in about 25%. Seizures, often generalized, occur in 25–35% and are more commonly associated with frontal lobe lesions. Focal neurologic deficits occur in 50%, with hemiparesis being the most common presentation.

In all patients with suspected brain abscess, a **computed tomography (CT) scan** should be obtained urgently. In addition, the paranasal sinuses, mastoids, and middle ear should be evaluated. A chest radiograph should be done to rule out suppurative lung lesions. CT is very sensitive for the diagnosis of brain abscess but is not specific, as neoplasms, granulomas, cerebral infarction, and resolving hematomas may give similar radiologic pictures. **Magnetic resonance imaging** (MRI) may better differentiate between an abscess collection and other conditions, and it has become the procedure of choice for this purpose.

Optimal management of brain abscesses usually includes both antibiotic therapy and surgical drainage, either through aspiration or complete excision. Progression of neurologic signs mandates emergent surgery. The antibiotic regimens most often recommended include high-dose penicillin or a third-generation cephalosporin, such as cefotaxime or cefuroxime, in combination with either metronidazole or chloramphenicol for greater anaerobic coverage. Corticosteroids often are used concomitantly in the management of raised intracranial pressure, and they do not appear to alter mortality rates. A total of 4–6 weeks of antimicrobial therapy is recommended, since there is no effective way to determine resolution of infection based on either CT or MRI findings, postoperatively.

In the present patient, the classic triad of headache, fever, and focal neurologic deficit suggested the diagnosis of brain abscess. The history of recurrent sinusitis made brain abscess even more likely. An emergent CT scan revealed pansinusitis and a left frontal hypodense lesion with uniform ring enhancement surrounding parenchymal edema. An urgent craniotomy was performed. Operative cultures revealed *Streptococcus viridans.* High-dose cefotaxime and metronidazole were prescribed and continued for 4 weeks, and the patient recovered with only mild residual weakness of the right lower extremity.

Clinical Pearls

1. The classic triad of fever, headache, and focal neurologic deficit suggests the diagnosis of brain abscess.

2. Paranasal sinusitis predisposes to frontal lobe abscess, whereas sphenoidal sinusitis predisposes to temporal lobe or sella turcica abscess. Otogenic abscesses typically are found in the temporal lobes.

3. *S. aureus* causes most cases of traumatic or postsurgical abscess. The remainder usually are polymicrobial, with various streptococci, enteric gram-negative bacilli, and anaerobes present.

4. Hemiparesis is the most common neurologic finding on presentation.

5. When a brain abscess is suspected, a lumbar puncture is contraindicated.

6. Treatment of pyogenic brain abscess includes broad-spectrum antibiotics, such as high-dose penicillin or a third-generation cephalosporin, in combination with metronidazole or chloramphenicol. Surgical drainage almost always is necessary.

REFERENCES

1. Wispelwey B, Scheld WM: Brain abscess: Etiology, diagnosis, and treatment. Infect Med 1990; 9:13.
2. Seydoux C, Francioli P: Bacterial brain abscesses: Factors influencing mortality and sequelae. Clin Infect Dis 1992;15:394–401.
3. Heilpern KL, Lorber B: Focal intracranial infections. Infect Dis Clin North Am 1996; 10:879–898.

PATIENT 47

A 39-year-old man with neutropenic leukemia, fever, and papular rash

A 39-year-old man with a history of acute myelogenous leukemia (AML) has been in the hospital for 14 days because of febrile neutropenia following his last chemotherapy. On admission, he was started on broad-spectrum antibiotic coverage with ceftazidime and gentamicin. All cultures were negative. After 2–3 days of therapy, he defervesced, but fever recurred on hospital day 7. After repeat cultures, vancomycin was added to the regimen. Over the past week, intermittent fever to 39.4°C has occurred, and the patient is complaining of rigors, myalgias, headache, and blurred vision in his right eye. He has noted several red lesions on his legs.

Physical Examination: Temperature 39.2°; pulse 114; respirations 16; blood pressure 110/65. General: ill appearing. HEENT: pupils equal, round, and reactive to light; extraocular muscles intact; fundi poorly visualized; tympanic membranes clear; oropharynx mildly injected; no ulcerations. Chest: clear to auscultation; infusaport device at upper right—site is nontender and nonerythematous. Cardiac: no murmur. Abdomen: soft, nontender, no organomegaly. Skin: erythematous papular lesions, nonblanching and nonpruritic, most notable on upper back and upper thighs (see figure); no perianal lesions.

Laboratory Findings: Hct 28%; WBC 400/μl (too few cells for differential); platelets 89,000/μl. Na$^+$ 136 mEq/L, K$^+$ 3.9 mEq/L, Cl$^-$ 112 mEq/L, HCO$_3^-$ 18 mEq/L. BUN 16 mg/dl, creatinine 1.2 mg/dl. Urinalysis: no cells present. Repeat blood cultures: no growth at 24 hours. Chest radiograph: normal.

Questions: What is the suspected diagnosis? What is the next step in managing this patient?

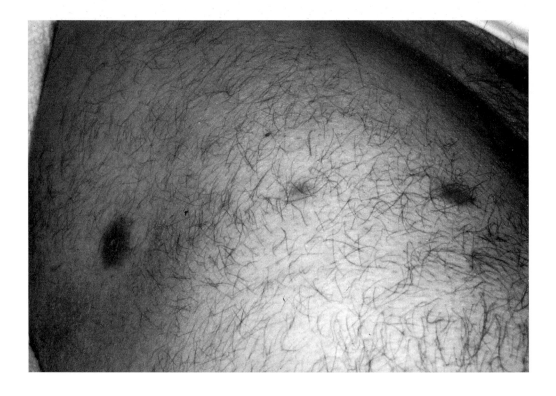

Answers: Disseminated candidiasis. Initiate treatment with amphotericin B.

Discussion: New skin lesions in a neutropenic patient can be manifestations of numerous cutaneous or systemic infections. Skin biopsy is indicated in all immunocompromised patients with new skin lesions to allow a rapid, potentially lifesaving diagnosis.

Characteristic skin lesions are found in 5–10% of patients with disseminated candidiasis. The lesions may be numerous or few in number; generalized or local in distribution; and papular, nodular, or pustular. Occasionally, the lesions of disseminated candidiasis may appear as purpura fulminans, echthyma gangrenosum, or a generalized erytroderma or macular rash, being easily confused with a cutaneous drug eruption. The organism can be cultured from 50% of skin biopsy specimens. Blood cultures usually are positive in patients with skin lesions, as opposed to the < 50% yield in patients without lesions. Skin lesions are found most frequently in disseminated disease caused by *C. tropicalis.*

In the neutropenic host, risk for invasive fungal infections is influenced by the severity and duration of neutropenia, the use of broad-spectrum antimicrobials (which alter the host's normal flora and permit overgrowth of *Candida* species), and the use of long-term intravascular devices. Disseminated *Candida* infection may involve multiple organ systems, with formation of microabscesses. Hepatosplenic involvement should be excluded since macroabscesses may form in these organs. Endophthalmitis can occur in 5–50% of neutropenic hosts, warranting a careful ophthalmalogic exam in all candidemic patients. The kidney, heart, gastrointestinal tract, and lung also are frequently involved.

Amphotericin B should be prescribed initially as empiric antifungal therapy in these patients because of the diversity of fungal pathogens responsible for disease. In most cases of candidemia and disseminated candidiasis, fluconazole is an effective alternative to amphotericin B.

In the present patient, recurrent fever while on broad-spectrum antibiotics strongly suggested the possibility of systemic fungal infection. A Gram stain of one of the lesions revealed budding yeast, and culture yielded *Candida tropicalis,* as did the blood cultures after 6-day incubation. Upon removal, the infusaport also yielded *C. tropicalis* on semiquantitative culture. Antifungal therapy with amphotericin B (1 mg/kg) was initiated, to a total cumulative dose of 1500 mg over the course of therapy. An ophthalmology evaluation revealed evidence of early endophthalmitis in his right eye. This was treated with intravitreous amphotericin B. CT scans during therapy and 3 months later revealed no evidence of hepatosplenic lesions. Six months later, his acute myelogenous leukemia remained in remission.

Clinical Pearls

1. The duration and severity of neutropenia, use of broad-spectrum antibiotics, and the presence of long-term vascular devices increase the risk of systemic fungal infections in the leukemic patient.

2. Cutaneous lesions occur in 5–10% of cases of disseminated candidiasis and are more commonly associated with *C. tropicalis* infections.

3. The responsible organism can be cultured from 50% of skin biopsy specimens.

4. Blood cultures usually are positive in patients with cutaneous lesions due to *Candida,* in contrast to the < 50% yield of blood cultures in patients without lesions.

REFERENCES
1. Bodey GP: Dermatologic manifestations of infections in neutropenic patients. Infect Dis Clin North Am 1994; 8:655–675.
2. Uzun O, Anaissie E: Problems and controversies in the management of hematogenous candidiasis. Clin Infect Dis 1996; 22(Suppl 2):95–99.
3. Walsh TS, Hiemenz JW, Anaissie E: Recent progress and current problems in treatment of invasive fungal infections in neutropenic patients. Infect Dis Clin North Am 1996; 10:365–400.

PATIENT 48

A 60-year-old man with bilateral pulmonary opacities

A 60-year-old man is admitted to the intensive care unit because of hypovolemic shock due to an acute diverticular hemorrhage. Intravenous crystaloid and blood products are administered, but persistent bleeding and hemodynamic instability after 48 hours necessitate an emergent right hemicolectomy. Four days postoperatively, the patient is hemodynamically stable and off vasopressor medications. However, prolonged mechanical ventilation is required because of underlying obstructive airway disease and electrolyte abnormalities. On day 5, he is noted to be more lethargic, tachypneic, and diaphoretic.

Physical Examination: Temperature 39.7°; pulse 114; respirations 28 (ventilator rate 10); blood pressure 100/50. General: confused and combative. Endotracheal tube: copious, mucopurulent secretions. Chest: coarse rhonchi auscultated in both lung fields. Cardiac: sinus tachycardia, no murmur. Neck: jugular veins not distended. Abdomen: incision is well approximated, no evidence of erythema or drainage. Extremities: mild acral cyanosis, no rash or peripheral edema.

Laboratory Findings: Hct 29%; WBC 15,800/μl with 79% neutrophils, 8% bands, 13% lymphocytes. Na^+ 130 mEq/L, K^+ 4.2 mEq/L, Cl^- 99 mEq/L, HCO_3^- 14 mEq/L. BUN 45 mg/dl, creatinine 2.2 mg/dl. Urinalysis: no cells. Arterial blood gas (FiO_2 0.40): pH 7.36, PCO_2 28 mmHg, PO_2 59 mmHg. Electrocardiogram: no acute ST-T wave changes. Sputum Gram stain: abundant WBC and gram-negative rods. Chest radiograph: see figure.

Question: What is the likely cause of this patient's pneumonia?

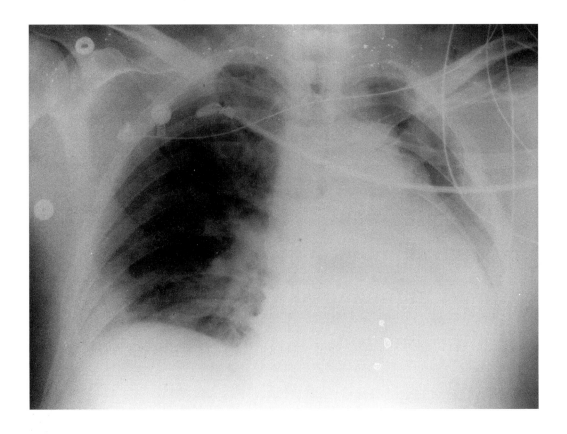

Diagnosis: Nosocomial pneumonia due to *Pseudomonas aeruginosa*

Discussion: *P. aeruginosa,* a gram-negative aerobic bacilli, is an important nosocomial pathogen and the leading cause of nosocomial pneumonia. Although sometimes present as part of the normal human flora, *P. aeruginosa* colonization increases markedly in hospitalized patients, especially those in an intensive care setting. Serious burns, mechanical ventilation, chemotherapeutic agents, and antibiotic therapy are important predisposing conditions for colonization and the subsequent potential for infection.

Lower respiratory tract infections occur almost exclusively in patients with compromised local respiratory or systemic host defenses. Congestive heart failure and chronic lung disease predisposes hospitalized patients to respiratory infections with nosocomial pathogens. Pulmonary infections due to *P. aeruginosa* generally do not occur in the community setting except in persons with specific risk factors for long-term colonization, such as underlying bronchiectasis or cystic fibrosis. Bacteremic *Pseudomonas* pneumonia occurs primarily in patients with hematologic malignancy or chemotherapy-induced neutropenia.

P. aeruginosa causes a fulminant, necrotizing pneumonia characterized by fever, chills, severe dyspnea, cyanosis, production of copious purulent sputum, and signs of severe systemic toxocity. Chest radiograph reveals a diffuse bronchopneumonia with distinct nodular opacities, correlating to areas of microabscess formation and alveolar necrosis (see figure). Cavitation typically is evident on chest radiograph within 48 hours of disease onset. Pleural effusions are common.

Because of the fulminant nature of *Pseudomonas* pneumonia, it usually is advisable to begin empiric antipseudomonal antibiotics in all cases of nosocomial pneumonia, especially in those patients with multiple risk factors for prior colonization. The use of two parenteral agents is preferred. Standard therapy includes a β-lactam agent, such as piperacillin or ceftazidime, and an antipseudomonal aminoglycoside. Alternative agents include imipenem/cilastin, aztreonam, or ciprofloxacin. If blood and sputum cultures reveal no pseudomonads, it generally is safe to switch to appropriate monotherapy.

The present patient's pneumonia slowly resolved on therapy with piperacillin and gentamicin, which were continued for 14 days. The patient was successfully extubated on day 10 of therapy, and subsequent recovery was uneventful.

Clinical Pearls

1. Risk factors for *P. aeruginosa* respiratory colonization and infection include hospitalization (especially in intensive care), mechanical ventilation, and previous antibiotic exposure. Bacteremia pneumonia occurs primarily in patients with hematologic malignancy or chemotherapy-induced neutropenia.

2. Underlying bronchiectasis or cystic fibrosis predisposes to long-term colonization with pseudomonads, with mucoid strains present in the latter condition.

3. Empiric therapy for nosocomial pneumonia generally should include two antipseudomonal agents. If *Pseudomonas* is not recovered from the respiratory tract, therapy can be tailored to appropriate monotherapy.

REFERENCES
1. Tillotson JR, Lerner AM: Characteristics of nonbacteremic Pseudomonas pneumonia. Ann Intern Med 1968; 68:295–307.
2. Karnad A, Alvarez S, Bok SL: Pneumonia caused by gram-negative bacilli. Am J Med 1985; 79:61.
3. Levison ME, Kaye D: Pneumonia caused by gram-negative bacilli: An overview. Rev Infect Dis 1985; 7:656–665.

PATIENT 49

A 10-year-old boy with fever, headache, and petechial rash

A 10-year old boy presents to the emergency department with a 3-day history of headache, chills, and fever after camping in rural Pennsylvania. Prior to these symptoms, he experienced nausea, vomiting, and abdominal pain for 2 days. He denies cough, chest pain, and diarrhea. He is penicillin-allergic.

Physical Examination: Temperature 40°; pulse 110; respirations 20; blood pressure 120/60. General: ill appearing. HEENT: periorbital edema, bilateral conjunctival suffusion. Cardiac: unremarkable. Chest: unremarkable. Abdomen: generalized tenderness, no rebound, no organomegaly. Extremities: edema on hands and feet, petechial rash on ankles and wrists (see figure).

Laboratory Findings: WBC 10,000/μl, platelets 160,000/μl. Aspartate aminotransferase: elevated 3X normal. Alkaline phosphatase: normal. Electrolytes: normal. BUN and creatinine: normal. Chest radiograph: unremarkable.

Question: What is the likely diagnosis?

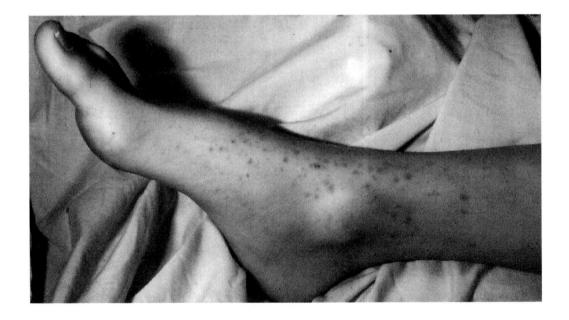

Diagnosis: Rocky Mountain spotted fever

Discussion: Rocky Mountain spotted fever (RMSF) is carried by the dog tick *Dermacentor variabilis*. The incubation period is 2–14 days, and the illness usually begins abruptly. Initial manifestation includes fever, headache, and severe myalgia. **Petechial rash** involves the wrist and ankles and typically is present 3–5 days after the clinical onset of illness. RMSF may present with prominent central nervous system or abdominal findings, and the clinician must be careful not to miss the rash in these patients. RMSF without spots is erlichiosis until proven otherwise.

Laboratory findings are not specific, but **thrombocytopenia** may be profound. The WBC count usually is normal or slightly increased. Liver function test results frequently increase. Anemia and azotemia are common accompaniments. Pulmonary findings are not present in the early phase, but patients may develop acute respiratory distress syndrome preterminally, due to pulmonary vasculitis. Patients with RMSF, therefore, have **negative chest radiographs** on initial clinical presentation. If an opacity is present, then an alternative diagnosis, such as atypical measles, should be entertained.

Physical findings include petechial rash, **conjunctival suffusion,** and **periorbital edema.** Dorsal **edema of the hands and feet** is another important clue and is seen in only a few other diseases (e.g., toxic shock syndrome and Kawasaki syndrome).

The diagnosis of RMSF is made by doing a Weil-Felix test using proteus OX-19 and OX-2 agglutination reaction alternately. Indirect hemaglutination titer of $\geq$ 1–128 is diagnostic in a patient with a compatible illness. Treatment is with chloramphenicol or doxycycline for 7–14 days. Erythromycin, aminoglycosides, trimethoprim-sulfamethoxazole, β-lactams, and quinolones are ineffective. If treated early and appropriately, RMSF usually is not fatal. Death due to RMSF occurs from myocarditis.

The present patient exhibited key symptoms of Rocky Mountain spotted fever, and his camping trip in a rural area made contact with ticks likely. A Weil-Felix test confirmed the diagnosis. He responded to doxycycline after 3 days and recovered fully after 14 days of treatment.

Clinical Pearls

1. Thrombocytopenia with normal WBC in a patient with petechial rash suggests Rocky Mountain spotted fever or meningococcemia.

2. The rash of RMSF begins on the ankles and wrists and extends centrally, in contrast to the rash of meningococcemia which has no particular pattern.

3. Central nervous system or abdominal symptoms may predominate on initial presentation and obscure the diagnosis of RMSF.

4. Conjunctival suffusion and periorbital edema are important clinical clues to RMSF, especially if found together with edema of the hands and feet.

5. Complications of RMSF include rhabdomyositis, acute respiratory distress syndrome, coagulopathy, and myocarditis.

REFERENCES
1. Weber DJ, Walker DH: Rocky Mountain spotted fever. Infect Dis Clin North Am 1991; 5:19–35.
2. Woodward TE: Rocky Mountain spotted fever: A present-day perspective. Medicine 1992; 71:255–259.
3. Kirkland KB, Marcom PK, Sexton DJ: Rocky Mountain spotted fever complicated by gangrene: Report of 6 cases and review. Clin Infect Dis 1993; 16:629–634.
4. Archibald LK, Sexton DJ: Long-term sequelae of Rocky Mountain spotted fever. Clin Infect Dis 1995; 20:1122–1125.
5. Walker DH: Rocky Mountain spotted fever: A seasonal alert. Clin Infect Dis 1995; 20:1111–1117.
6. Woodward TE: Remember Rocky Mountain spotted fever: A lesson in ethical principles. Clin Infect Dis 1996; 23:165–166.

PATIENT 50

A 58-year-old man with fever post coronary artery bypass graft surgery

The patient is a 58-year-old man with a 17-year history of coronary artery disease who managed successfully medically until unstable angina developed. He underwent coronary angiography, which revealed minimal disease, and coronary bypass surgery. Postoperatively, antihypertensive and antianginal medications were continued, and docusate sodium (Colace) was started. His past medical history is significant for hypertensive cholesteremia and hypertension. He is a social drinker and has been a heavy smoker for 30 years. His family history is positive for coronary artery disease.

Physical Examination (Preoperative):   Temperature 37.2°; pulse 82; respirations 14, blood pressure 220/110. General: obese, no acute distress. HEENT: grade II hypertensive changes; carotid bruits present, but no jugular venous distinction. Cardiac: no interstitial signs, soft S_1 murmur and left-sided S_4, left renal bruit. Abdomen: no organomegaly, no hepatojugular reflex. Extremities: statis dermatitis of lower legs.

Hospital Course: Coronary artery bypass graft (CABG) surgery uneventful; postoperative period normal until fever developed on day 7. Temperature 40.5°, pulse 90. General: *not* acutely ill appearing; physical exam unrevealing except for slight discharge from vein graft site on leg. Chest radiographs: questionable left lobe opacity with definite small, left-sided pleural effusion. WBC 19,800/μl with 62% polymorphonuclear cells, 4% bands, 6% eosinophils, and 18% lymphocytes; platelets normal; ESR 110 mm/hr. Urinalysis: RBC 5/hpf, WBC 0/hpf. Liver function and renal function tests: normal. Blood cultures: negative. Leg wound culture: *Citrobacter freundii.* Urine cultures: *Stentophomonas maltophilia.*

Question: What condition is suggested by the patient's clinical presentation?

Diagnosis: Drug fever

Discussion: Septic complications from CABG surgery are infrequent. When they do occur, they usually are skin or soft tissue infections, rather than infections of the sternal or leg wounds. Mediastinitis and sternal osteomyelitis are rare complications of CABG. Similarly, nosocomial urinary tract infections are relatively uncommon in this setting. Patients may, however, develop nosocomial pneumonia.

In this patient, a wound infection is an unlikely explanation for the fever because the wound description is not impressive. The organism that grew from the leg wound exudate—a common site for colonization—was *Citrobacter freundii,* an infrequent pathogen in this setting. There is no sternal tenderness or instability to suggest sternal osteomyelitis. The chest radiograph does not suggest mediastinitis. The minimal opacity seen in the left lower lobe probably reports basal atelectasis, which commonly follows this type of surgery. Likewise, left-sided pleural effusion is normally found following open heart surgery. Therefore, although the chest radiograph is not normal, it does not suggest nosocomial pneumonia. The urinalysis reveals no white cells, but *Stentophomonas maltophilia* grew from culture of the urine. This combination of findings suggests colonization, rather than infection, of the urinary tract and should not be considered as a cause of the patient's fever.

Symptoms still unaccounted for include temperature elevation, pulse temperature deficit, elevated WBC, and eosinophilia. An elevated ESR is regularly associated with a major surgical procedure and is not helpful in this situation. The most important diagnostic clues are **relative bradycardia** (see figure) and the presence of **eosinophilia** in a patient who does not appear acutely ill. This constellation of findings suggests a drug fever as the cause of the patient's temperature elevation.

While the patient's antihypertensive medications are a common cause of drug fever, Colace is the more likely culprit. **Colace** contains sulfur—**a common cause of drug fever** in hospitalized patients. Treatment consists of discontinuing the medication, and the fever almost always resolves in 72 hours.

The present patient had a drug fever due to the sulfur components of his stool softener, Colace. The combination of relative bradycardia and eosinophilia was the clue to the diagnosis. The Colace was discontinued, and the fever resolved within 3 days.

Clinical Pearls

1. Most patients with drug fever have an atopic history and look "inappropriately well" for the degree of fever.

2. All patients with drug fever and a temperature of $\geq 39°C$ (without arrythmias, pacemaker, or β-blocker medication) will have relative bradycardia.

3. Eosinophils almost always are present early in the course of drug fever, but eosinophilia is uncommon.

4. Serum transaminases are mildly elevated early in the course of drug fever. ESR may be ≥ 100 mm/hr.

REFERENCES
1. Hanson MA: Drug fever: Remember to consider it in diagnosis. Postgrad Med 1991; 89:167–170.
2. Johnson DH, Cunha BA: Drug fever. Infect Dis Clin North Am 1996; 10:85–92.

PATIENT 51

A 30-year-old man with erythematous rash vacationing in eastern Long Island

A 30-year-old man returns from vacationing on eastern Long Island in the Hamptons and presents to the hospital with sore throat, neck stiffness, and an erythematous, circular rash on the back. The patient spent his vacation at the beach and did not recall being bitten by a tick. Symptoms of malaise and low-grade fever developed several days prior to admission and before the rash appeared. He complains of no other skin lesions and notes that the rash is warm, but not painful or itchy. He initially thought that it was an insect bite and did not seek medical attention until the other symptoms developed. The patient has been in good health and denies cough, chest pain, and abdominal pain. Past medical history is positive for hypercholesterolemia and a tonsillectomy in childhood.

Physical Examination: Temperature 38.7°; pulse 68; respirations 12; blood pressure 110/70. General: well appearing. HEENT: fundi unremarkable. Chest: no abnormal sounds. Cardiac: normal S_1S_2; no murmurs, gallops, or clicks. Skin: erythematous, annular rash on back (see figure). Musculoskeletal: no costovertebral angle tenderness or spinal tenderness. Extremities: no pedal edema, no rashes.

Laboratory Examination: Hct 36%; WBC 8300/µl with 66% polymorphonuclear cells, 4% monocytes, 30% lymphocytes. ESR 22 mm/hr; transaminases elevated 1.5X normal. Alkaline-phosphatase: normal. BUN and creatinine: normal. Electrocardiogram: incomplete right bundle branch block. Chest radiograph: questionable hilar adenopathy.

Question: What is the most likely diagnosis based on this presentation?

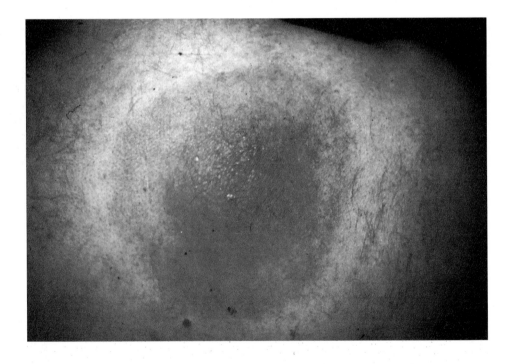

Diagnosis: Erythema migrans due to Lyme disease

Discussion: Lyme disease occurs in most areas of the United States, but is particularly prevalent in the Northwest and Northeast. It is transmitted by the *Ixodes* tick, and the causative agent is *Borrelia burgdorferi*. Many patients do not recall a history of tick bite. This is probably because *Ixodes* ticks in the Northeast and upper Midwest and *Ixodes pacificus* ticks along the western coast of the U.S. are tiny and, therefore, barely noticeable.

The disease may be divided into three distinct clinical stages: stage 1 is characterized by erythema migrans; stage 2 features neurologic and cardiac involvement; and stage 3 is characterized by Lyme arthritis. It should be appreciated that the stages represent a continuum; nevertheless, they do allow classification of the disease. Importantly, erythema migrans (EM) is observable in only 50–75% of patients. It usually develops 2 weeks after the tick bite, but may develop as late as 3 weeks after the tick bite. Systemic symptoms, such as **fever, malaise, stiff neck, fatigue, or headache**, usually occur concurrently.

Hematologic dissemination of *Borrelia* is characterized clinically by multiple EM lesions, fever, arthralgias, and meningismus within the first few weeks of infection. Meningitis, myocarditis (with or without AV conduction abnormalities), and abnormal liver function tests also may be seen early in Lyme disease. There are few disorders that can be confused with this disease entity. Ringworm is one, but generally it can be differentiated by its association with intense pruritis. Alternately, multifocal EM lesions may be confused with erythema multiforme. Erythema multiforme lesions tend to be more numerous and smaller; it is unusual to see more than a dozen skin lesions in Lyme disease.

The presence of erythema migrans rash is diagnostic for Lyme disease, making a Lyme serology unnecessary. If a Lyme serology had been obtained at the time of presentation in this case, it most likely would have been negative. When necessary (i.e., the patient does not have the rash, but Lyme disease is suspected clinically), an IgM titer should be obtained 6–8 weeks after the presumed time of infection. After 6–8 weeks, the IgM titer is elevated, and the IgG is normal—unless there has been prior exposure to the spirochete. Over the next several months, the IgM titer gradually decreases, and the IgG titer increases. It is important to realize that after 6 months the IgM titer should be negative. The IgG titer will remain elevated with fluctuations for life.

After a period of 6–12 months, if a patient has symptoms compatible with Lyme disease, a positive titer does not imply a causal relationship but a negative IgG titer effectively rules out Lyme disease as a diagnostic consideration. Most patients with EM can be treated with a 2-week course of either amoxicillin or doxycycline. Note that there is no evidence to suggest that treating stage 1 Lyme disease for longer than 2 weeks has any benefit. Macrolides are second-line therapy. A macrolide may be used in children or pregnant women who are penicillin-allergic.

The present patient had classic EM, as evidenced by the erythema migrans rash on his back. He was given oral doxycycline, with good results. Chronic complications did not develop.

Clinical Pearls

1. Erythema migrans is diagnostic of Lyme disease, making serologic testing unnecessary.

2. When Lyme serology is ordered, IgM and IgG determinations should be done separately and not combined or expressed as a ratio.

3. IgM antibodies rise 6–8 weeks after infection and peak within 6 months. IgG titers begin rising after a few months and remain elevated with fluctuations for life.

4. Elevated IgM titers suggest active clinical disease, whereas elevated IgG titers do not correlate with clinical disease and usually indicate past exposure to the antigen.

5. Optimal treatment of ECM is 2 weeks of either oral amoxicillin or doxycycline. In penicillin-intolerant children and pregnant females, a macrolide may be used.

REFERENCES
1. Dennis DT: Lyme disease. Dermatol Clin 1995;13:537–551.
2. Nocton JJ, Steere AC: Lyme disease. Adv Med 1995; 40:69–117.
3. Coyle PK: Advances and pitfalls in the diagnosis of Lyme disease. FEMS Immunol Med Microbiol 1997; 19:103–109.
4. Evans J: Lyme disease. Curr Opin Rheumatol 1997; 9:328–336.

PATIENT 52

A 48-year-old man with headache, myalgia, and cough

A 48-year-old man presents with a 6-day history of progressive headache, myalgia, and nonproductive cough. On admission his headaches are severe and frontal in location, and he appears moderately ill. An earlier chest radiograph had revealed a dense, left lower lobe opacity. The patient denies shaking chills, night sweats, and chest or abdominal pain. Past medical history is significant for a cholecystectomy 10 years ago and a right total knee replacement (due to osteoarthritis) 2 years ago. The patient has no known allergies. He is the owner of a pet shop.

Physical Examination: Temperature 39.8°; pulse 100; respirations 22; blood pressure 190/88. General: moderately ill-appearing and coughing. HEENT: approximately six nontender, nonpruritic, and nonblanching macules on the forehead and face. Chest: left lower lobe rales. Cardiac: S_1S_2 unremarkable, S_4 present, II/VI systolic ejection murmur heard at apex. Abdomen: soft, nontender, no bruits; questionable hepatomegaly; no splenomegaly. Extremities: no edema or rash.

Laboratory Findings: WBC 18,200/μl with a left shift. Creatinine 1.9 mg/dl, BUN 28 mg/dl. Urinalysis: 1+ proteinuria, WBC 0/hpf, RBC 2/hpf. Alkaline phosphatase: normal. Aspartate aminotransferase: 2× normal. Chest radiograph: left lower lobe opacity, no effusion or cavitation, no hilar adenopathy (see figure).

Question: Based on the patient's presentation and subsequent work-up, what is the most likely diagnosis?

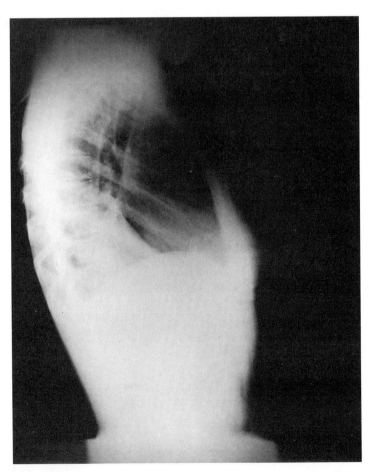

Diagnosis: Psittacosis

Discussion: Psittacosis is a disease caused by *Chlamydia psittaci* that is transmitted from psittacine birds to humans by droplet infection. Psittacosis is one of the **zoonotic atypical pneumonias** suggested by a history of contact with psittacine birds. Psittacosis presents with severe headache, myalgia, and nonspecific respiratory symptoms. As with other atypical pneumonias, psittacosis is a systemic infectious disease, and clues to its presence are based on **extrapulmonary manifestations.**

The presence of a pulse-temperature deficit (relative bradycardia) in a patient with atypical pneumonia limits diagnostic possibilities to psittacosis, Q fever, or legionnaires' disease. A macular rash, called **Horder's spots**, is characteristic of psittacosis. Horder's spots resemble the rose spots of typhoid fever, but are on the face in psittacosis, rather than on the abdomen. Additional features suggesting psittacosis are hepatic tenderness or enlargement and mild elevations of the serum transaminases.

Confirmation of the diagnosis is made retrospectively by serologic means. The tube agglutination test usually shows a fourfold or greater rise between acute and convalescent titers. Early empiric antimicrobial therapy may delay or eliminate the titer rise. Preferred treatment for psittacosis is **doxycycline**; macrolides are less effective. Treatment ordinarily is continued for 10–14 days.

The present patient's exposure in a pet shop, physical symptoms including rash, and mildly elevated serum transaminases led to a diagnosis of psittacosis. Serologic tests confirmed this suspicion. He was treated with doxycycline for 2 weeks, with gradual resolution of the left lower lobe opacity. The patient had a full and uneventful recovery.

Clinical Pearls

1. Psittacosis, tularemia, and Q fever are zoonotic pneumonias.

2. Horder's spots, which resemble the rose spots of typhoid fever but are found on the face, are the cutaneous manifestation of psittacosis.

3. Psittacosis is associated with a pulse-temperature deficit (relative bradycardia) and liver involvement, which usually is manifested as mild-to-moderate increases in the serum transaminases.

4. Obscure phlebitis is a recognized complication during the convalescent period following psittacosis.

REFERENCES
1. Oldach DW, Gaydos CA, Mundy LM, et al: Rapid diagnosis of *Chlamydia psittaci* pneumonia. Clin Infect Dis 1993; 17:338–343.
2. Cunha BA, Ortega AM: Atypical pneumonias. Postgrad Med 1996; 99:123–132.
3. Gregory DW, Schaffner W: Psittacosis. Semin Respir Ther 1997; 12:7–11.

PATIENT 53

A 40-year-old woman with fever and eosinophilia

A 40-year-old woman presents with a 2-week history of fever and myalgia. She noted nausea and diarrhea during the first week of her illness, both of which resolved spontaneously. The patient also reports bilateral periorbital edema associated with tenderness in the masseter. She denies cough, chest pain, night sweats, and rashes. She has no known allergies, and her medical history is significant for diabetes mellitus.

Physical Examination: Temperature 38.6°; pulse 110; respirations 18; blood pressure 190/84. General: well-appearing. HEENT: bilateral periorbital edema and bilateral conjunctival hemorrhages (see figure). Cardiac: unremarkable. Abdomen: soft, nontender, no organomegaly. Extremities: subungual splinter hemorrhages bilaterally on hands and feet.

Laboratory Findings: WBC 9800/µl with 82% neutrophils, 8% lymphocytes, 10% eosinophils; platelets normal; ESR 2 mm/hr. BUN and creatinine: normal. Liver function tests: normal. Aspartate aminotransferase: 2× normal. Creatine phosphokinase: 12× normal. Chest radiograph: negative. Blood cultures: negative.

Question: What is the explanation for this patient's presentation?

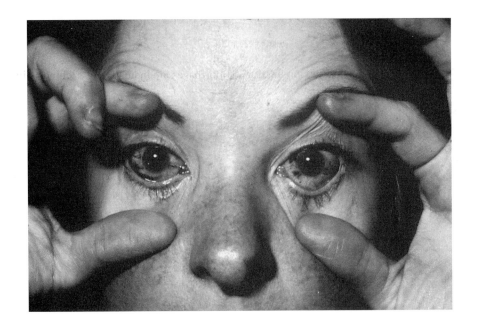

Diagnosis: Trichinosis

Discussion: Humans are the incidental host of *Trichinella spiralis*. Disease commonly results from eating undercooked pork from an animal that has ingested garbage contaminated with *Trichinella*. *Trichinella* also surfaces after eating contaminated, undercooked bear, walrus, horse, or wild boar meat.

Clinical symptoms depend on larvae inoculum. Symptoms usually begin 1 week after infestation, with nausea, vomiting, and diarrhea. The diarrhea is caused by the adult worms migrating through the intestine. During the second week, the larvae invade the muscles of multiple organs. Common symptoms after the second week include myositis with pain and swelling of arm and leg muscles. The periorbital muscles are involved early and manifest clinically as periorbital edema.

Bilateral subconjunctival hemorrhages are an important clue to the diagnosis. Some patients develop a maculopapular rash. Subungual splinter or retinal hemorrhages are not uncommon. Clinical diagnosis usually is straightforward in a patient with fever, myositis, periorbital edema, and subconjunctival hemorrhage. An ESR approaching zero coupled with eosinophilia is another important clue. Muscle biopsy usually is unnecessary, and an elevated bentonite flocculation titer establishes the diagnosis.

The present patient remembered eating a dinner of pork about 3 weeks previously while attending an event. Her physical symptoms, especially periorbital edema and conjunctival and subungual hemorrhages, as well as her ESR of 2 with eosinophilia strongly suggested trichinosis. An elevated bentonite flocculation titer confirmed the diagnosis. The patient's illness resolved without treatment after 4 weeks.

Clinical Pearls

1. The combination of myositis, eosinophilia, and a very low ESR suggests the diagnosis of trichinosis.

2. Gastrointestinal symptoms (i.e., nausea, vomiting, diarrhea) occur during the first week of illness (about 1 week after infection), and systemic signs occur after the second week.

3. Periorbital edema and subconjunctival hemorrhages are indicative of trichinosis in a patient with myositis.

REFERENCES

1. McAuley JB, Michelson MK, Schantz PM: Trichinella infection in travelers. J Infect Dis 1991; 164:1013–1016.
2. Mawhorter SD, Kazura JW: Trichinosis of the central nervous system. Semin Neurol 1993; 13:148–152.
3. Morse JW, Ridenour R, Unterseher P: Trichinosis: Infrequent diagnosis or frequent misdiagnosis? Ann Emerg Med 1994; 24:969–971.

PATIENT 54

An 18-year-old man with fever, headache, and rash

An 18-year-old student home on spring break from college presents to the emergency department with a 2-day history of low-grade fevers, runny nose, and increasing headache. Today, a stiff neck and petechial rash also developed. He is agitated, is experiencing photophobia, and has some difficulty hearing. He denies chest pain, abdominal pain, cough, diarrhea, and night sweats. The patient had an appendectomy as a child and is allergic to sulfonamides.

Physical Examination:　Temperature 39.6°; pulse 122; respirations 20; blood pressure 130/80. General: sick appearing, uncooperative. HEENT: fundi could not be visualized. Chest: clear. Cardiac: normal S_1S_2; no murmurs, gallops, rub, snaps, or clicks. Abdomen: no hepatosplenomegaly, nontender. Back: no costovertebral angle tenderness, some tenderness over lower back. Extremities: petechiae asymmetrically over upper and lower extremities, no purpuric lesions (see figure).

Laboratory Findings:　WBC 14,700/μl with 81% neutrophils, 12% lymphocytes, 7% monocytes; ESR 19 mm/hr. Liver function tests: unremarkable. BUN and creatinine: normal. Electrocardiogram: sinus tachycardia. Chest radiograph: no opacities or effusions. Cerebrospinal fluid (CSF): opening pressure increased, appearance cloudy. Gram stain: negative. Protein: slightly increased. Glucose: decreased. Lactic acid: 14 mg/dl.

Question:　What diagnosis is suggested by the patient's clinical presentation?

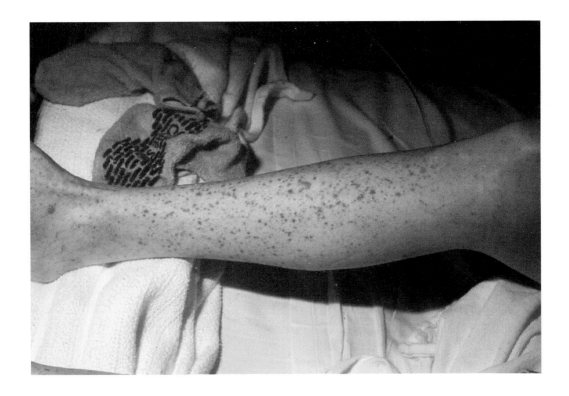

Diagnosis: Meningococcemia with meningococcal meningitis

Discussion: *Neisseria meningitidis* is a catalase-positive, oxidase-negative, gram-negative diplococcus that resides in the oropharynx. There are nine different meningococcal serotypes based on their polysaccharide capsules. The serotypes A, B, C, Y, and W135 are most commonly associated with clinical infection. The organisms are fastidious and grow best in the presence of an enhanced CO_2 atmosphere on chocolate agar or Thayer-Martin medium. *N. meningitides* requires only a few days for incubation, during which time patients have nonspecific upper respiratory tract symptoms. When the clinical disease presents, however, it is fulminant: death may ensue within a few hours.

Patients infected by *N. meningitides* have variable degrees of headache and myalgia which are nonspecific, and **early deafness** is a sign of many types of bacterial meningitis. Characteristically, petechial lesions are spread over the body. They are small initially, but enlarge over time and may become purpuric. The **number of petechial lesions correlates roughly with prognosis**—the more lesions there are, the more likely the disease will prove fatal. The meningococcemia may exist alone with only the acute febrile illness and rash, or may coexist with meningococcal meningitis. Moreover, meningococcal meningitis may present clinically without signs of meningococcemia.

CSF examination usually reveals a pleocytosis, with a gram stain positive for pleomorphic gram-negative diplococci. Occasionally, the CSF is turbid, and the Gram stain is negative. In this situation the most likely organism is the meningococcus, which presents with an acute bacterial meningitis, a negative Gram stain, and a cloudy CSF. In most cases, the organism can be demonstrated by Gram stain or culture of the fluid aspirated from petechial lesions.

The treatment of meningococcemia in meningitis is high-dose penicillin. Alternately, a third-generation cephalosporin in meningeal doses or chloramphenicol is effective.

In the present patient, the prodrome was typical and practically indistinguishable from a respiratory virus infection until high fever, stiff neck, and rash developed. The diagnosis was confirmed by blood cultures and CSF positive for *N. meningitides*. Meningococcemia and meningococcal meningitis were coexisting, a common clinical presentation. The patient was treated with high-dose, intravenous penicillin. He recovered with no sequelae.

Clinical Pearls

1. Meningococcemia may occur alone or with meningococcal meningitis. Meningococcal meningitis may exist alone, as well.

2. Cloudy CSF and a negative Gram stain are most frequently associated with *Neisseria meningitidis*.

3. Meningococcemia with meningococcal meningitis is one of the most rapidly fatal infectious diseases. Classically, patients are "well at 12 o'clock and dead by 3 o'clock." Early empiric treatment is essential.

4. The Waterhouse-Friderichsen syndrome (adrenal insufficiency and shock) results from adrenal invasion by the meningococcus in patients with meningococcemia.

REFERENCES
1. Sippel JE, Girgis NI, Kilpatrick ME, Farid Z: Laboratory diagnosis of bacterial meningitis. Trans R Soc Trop Med Hyg 1991; 85(Suppl 1):6–8.
2. Gottesman G, Israele V, Zierk-Diamond K, Salzman MB: Outcome of untreated meningococcal meningitis. Pediatr Infect Dis J 1996; 15:1048–1049.
3. Meningococcal meningitis. Weekly Epidemiol Record 1996; 71:103–104.

PATIENT 55

A 23-year-old woman with fever and headache

A 23-year-old woman returned 2 weeks ago from a tour in Latin America with the Peace Corps. She has not been feeling well since her arrival in the United States. She complains of fever with chills, headache, and malaise. She also notes intermittent, mild, right lower quadrant pain. She denies cough, chest pain, nightsweats, and diarrhea. Past medical history is significant for three episodes of infectious diarrhea during her tour in Latin America. The Peace Corps informed her that these episodes were due to *Shigella* on two occasions and *Campylobacter* on another. Prior to her return home, she travelled through several countries along the Amazon basin.

The patient sustained a traumatic fracture of her arm while playing hockey in high school, but otherwise has been in good health. She has no known allergies.

Physical Examination: Temperature 39.4; pulse 108; respirations 14; blood pressure 132/68. General: ill-appearing, with a blank stare. HEENT: unremarkable. Chest: clear. Cardiac: normal S_1S_2; no gallops, rubs, or clicks. Abdomen: questionable right lower quadrant pain; no hepatosplenomegaly, bruits, or fluid; six small, pink-colored macules on anterior abdominal wall. Extremities: no edema or rash.

Laboratory Examination: WBC 4600/μl with 66% polymorphonuclear cells, 5% bands, 29% lymphocytes; platelets 80,000/μl. BUN 124 mg/dl, creatinine 1.3 mg/dl. Urinalysis: WBC 0/hpf, RBC 0/hpf, 1+ protein, 1+ ketones. Liver function tests: aspartate aminotransferase 1.5× normal. Alkaline phosphatase: normal. Chest radiograph: no opacities or cardiac abnormalities. Plain film: normal gas pattern with generalized adynamic ileus (see figure). Stool cultures and blood cultures: pending. Malarial smears: negative.

Question: What is the most probable diagnosis?

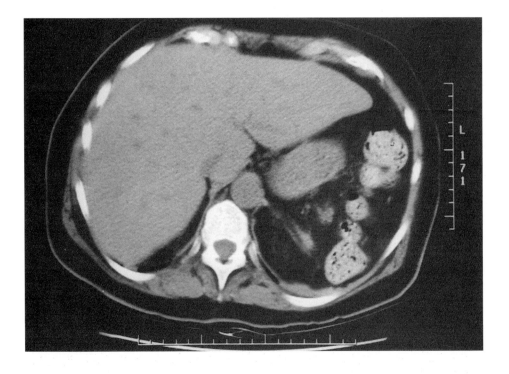

Diagnosis: Enteric fever caused by *Salmonella* infection

Discussion: The syndrome of enteric fever may be caused by *Salmonella typhi* as well as non-typhi salmonellae that invade the bloodstream and cause systemic disease. Patients with typhoid fever usually present with **characteristic apathetic facies and no localizing signs**. This latter feature makes diagnosis difficult before culture results are available.

Salmonellae are intracellular, gram-negative, aerobic organisms. Blood cultures typically are positive early in the illness. Subsequently, stool cultures become positive as the disease progresses. Note that **constipation**, rather than diarrhea, is the usual presenting symptom in typhoid fever, although diarrhea may later ensue. Patients with typhoid fever also complain of a **severe headache** and may have a mild, **nonproductive cough**, which tends to lead the unwary physician away from the correct diagnosis. If an early diagnosis is imperative, a biopsy of the bone marrow or liver usually reveals the presence of *Salmonella*.

An additional clinical clue to the presence of *Salmonella*-induced enteric fever is a pulse-temperature deficit, especially when accompanied by **relative bradycardia and leukopenia**.

Diagnosis of typhoid fever is by recovery of the organism from blood, stool, or other body fluid (e.g., bone marrow, liver biopsy specimen). Serologically, a single blood sample with an O titer $\geq$ 320 or an H antibody $\geq$ 640 is diagnostic of typhoid fever in a patient with typical clinical features.

The preferred empiric treatment of enteric fever caused by *Salmonella* is with a quinolone. Alternate appropriate therapies include trimethoprim-sulfamethoxazole, third-generation cephalosporins, doxycycline, or a carbapenem. Treatment ordinarily is continued for 10–14 days.

The present patient's relative bradycardia in concert with leukopenia was helpful in limiting differential diagnostic possibilities to typhoid fever and malaria. Both illnesses have much in common. Fortunately, in this case the patient had rose spots on her anterior abdomen, which was a clue to the diagnosis. Stool cultures were negative initially, but the blood cultures grew *Salmonella typhi*. She was treated with a quinolone for 2 weeks and had no complications of typhoid fever.

Clinical Pearls

1. Enteric fever due to *Salmonella* infection is an acute febrile illness, usually without localizing signs. The presence of rose spots suggests the possibility of typhoid fever.

2. Headache, apathetic facies, and a mild, nonproductive cough are characteristic presenting symptoms.

3. Leukopenia and relative bradycardia in the appropriate clinical setting suggest the diagnosis.

4. Constipation rather than diarrhea is the predominant mode of *S. typhi* presentation with enteric fever.

5. Optimal therapy is with a quinolone. Ampicillin should not be used because of the high prevalence of resistant strains.

REFERENCES
1. Durani AB, Rab SM: Changing spectrum of typhoid. J Pakistani Med Assoc 1996; 46:50–52.
2. Alsoub H, Uwaydah AK, Matar I, et al: A clinical comparison of typhoid fever caused by susceptible and multidrug-resistant strains of *Salmonella typhi*. Br J Clin Pract 1997; 51:8–10.
3. Rowe B, Ward LR, Threlfall EJ: Multidrug-resistant *Salmonella typhi:* A worldwide epidemic. Clin Infect Dis 1997; 24(Suppl 1):S106–S109.
4. Sood R, Roy S, Kaushik P: Typhoid fever with severe pancytopenia. Postgrad Med J 1997; 73:41–42.

PATIENT 56

A 50-year-old man with fever and left upper quadrant pain

A 50-year-old man presents with a 2-week history of fever following his chemotherapy treatment for acute myelogenous leukemia (AML). His temperature has been 38.9°C and he has experienced shaking chills for the previous 3 days. The patient denies cough, chest pain, headache, myalgia, and diarrhea. His past medical history is significant only for AML, diagnosed 7 months ago.

Physical Examination: Temperature 39.6; pulse 122; respirations 20; blood pressure 130/84. General: ill-appearing. HEENT: no abnormalities. Chest: no adventitious sounds bilaterally. Cardiac: normal, except gratuitous 1/6 systolic murmurs at apex. Abdomen: left upper quadrant tenderness, questionable splenomegaly, no hepatomegaly. Extremities: unremarkable.

Laboratory Findings: WBC 800/μl, numerous blasts noted; platelets decreased; ESR 55 mm/hr. Chest radiograph: no opacities seen. Liver function tests: alkaline phosphatase 4× normal. Aspartate and alanine aminotransferases: normal. BUN and creatinine: normal. Blood cultures: pending.

Question: How would you diagnose this patient?

Diagnosis: Hepatosplenic candidiasis

Discussion: Hepatosplenic candidiasis usually occurs in patients with acute leukemia after prolonged leukopenia from cancer chemotherapy. Leukopenic patients frequently have low-grade fever in spite of broad-spectrum antibiotic treatment. The fever heralds invasive fungal infection, which usually occurs after 2 weeks of profound neutropenia while the patient is on double-drug antipseudomonal coverage. Hepatosplenic candidiasis presents in this fashion and is clearly distinguishable by left upper quadrant pain. Hepatosplenic candidiasis is a manifestation of invasive, disseminated *Candida* in immunocompromised hosts. Therefore, other signs of disseminated candidiasis may be seen (e.g., candidal endopthalmitis) but usually are absent in these patients. An important laboratory clue to support the diagnosis is the finding of alkaline phosphatase elevation in a leukopenic host with left upper quadrant pain. These signs in a neutropenic cancer patient also suggest the diagnosis of hepatosplenic candidasis.

The diagnosis is confirmed by obtaining an abdominal ultrasound or computed tomography (CT) scan. These tests usually show multiple defects in the spleen and liver, which represent candidal abscesses. Such findings in a patient with positive blood cultures for *Candida* are diagnostic. Alternatively, a liver mass may be aspirated percutaneously under CT scan guidance and the aspirated material cultured.

Treatment is with fluconazole, which has been shown to achieve results superior to those obtained with amphotericin. Treatment should be continued until the liver and spleen masses resolve on CT scan and the alkaline phosphatase normalizes.

In the present patient, alkaline phosphatase elevation and left upper quadrant pain in the setting of AML and neutropenia narrowed the diagnosis to hepatosplenic candidiasis. CT scan revealed candidal abscesses (see figure, *arrows*), and blood cultures were positive for *Candida*. He was given fluconazole for 3 weeks, with complete recovery of lesions as evidenced by repeat CT scan of the abdomen.

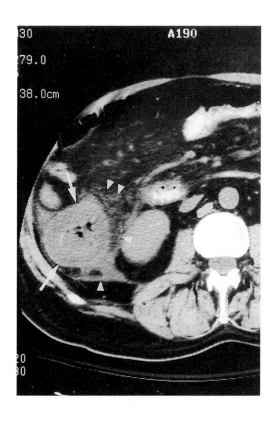

Clinical Pearls

1. Left upper quadrant pain and elevated alkaline phosphatase in a patient with prolonged fever and neutropenia are indicative of hepatosplenic candidiasis.

2. Candidal abscess of liver and spleen in hepatosplenic candidiasis are demonstrated by abdominal ultrasound or CT scan.

3. Fluconazole is superior to amphotericin B in the treatment of hepatosplenic candidiasis. Treatment should be continued until the lesions resolve.

REFERENCES

1. von Eiff M, Essink M, Roos N, et al: Hepatosplenic candidiasis: A late manifestation of Candida septicaemia in neutropenic patients with haematologic malignancies. Blut 1990; 60:242–248.
2. Loeliger A, van Leeuwen M, Rozenberg-Arska M, Dekker AW: Hepatosplenic candidiasis: A fatal disease? Infection 1992; 20:336–338.
3. Dear A: Hepatosplenic candidiasis in patients with acute leukemia: What is the optimum prophylaxis following subsequent chemotherapy? Eur J Haematol 1994; 52:184–186.

PATIENT 57

A 25-year old woman with erythematous hand swelling

A 25-year-old woman presents with an erythematous swelling on her hands that developed 1 week prior to admission. She is a school teacher, and she relates her skin condition to an ecology course that requires frequent contact with soil and water from local lakes and streams. She denies cough, chest pain, night sweats, and rashes. She states that the patches are warm and painful, but not pruritic. Past medical history includes an allergy to sulfonamides and diabetes mellitus managed successfully with oral hypoglycemics. The patient has been taking oral cefalexin for a week, with no effect on the lesions.

Physical Examination: Temperature 38.6°; pulse 110; respirations 12; blood pressure 180/72. HEENT: a few microaneurysms seen on retinal exam, otherwise no abnormalities noted. Cardiac: unremarkable. Abdomen: no organomegaly, normal bowel sounds, soft, nontender. Extremities: normal except for hand lesions that are warm to touch and poorly demarcated, 2-cm, erythematous papules on the arms (see figure). Lymph nodes: no evidence of lymphangitis; axillary and antecubital adenopathy bilaterally.

Laboratory Findings: Hct 40%; WBC 12,300/μl with 90% neutrophils (no left shift); platelets 240,000/μl. ESR 80 mm/hr, hemoglobin 14 g/dl, glucose 270 mg/dl. Alkaline phosphatase and aspartate aminotransferase: normal. Urinalysis: unremarkable. Chest radiograph: normal. Blood cultures: negative.

Question: What diagnosis should be considered given the features of this patient's presentation?

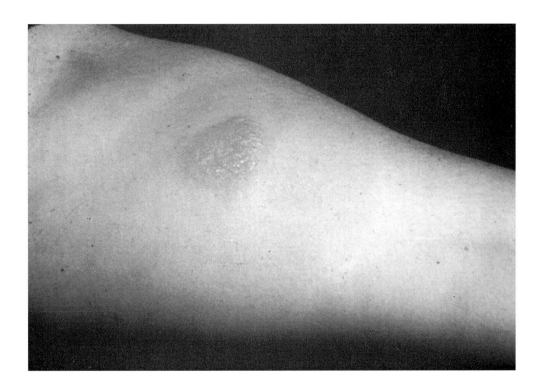

Diagnosis: Sweet's syndrome

Discussion: Sweet's syndrome is an idiopathic disorder that usually occurs in women and occasionally is associated with acute myelogenous leukemia. Typical presentation is an abrupt onset of tender, erythematous nodules on the extremities or a portion of the trunk, uniformly accompanied by fever. A leukocytosis with a left shift and an elevated ESR are characteristic of the syndrome.

The major criteria for the diagnosis of Sweet's syndrome are the presence of **painful, culture-negative, erythematous papules or pustules** with a **neutrophilic infiltration** of the skin, particularly in association with immune disorders, hematologic malignancies, or pregnancy. Leukocytoclastic vasculitis is *not* a feature. Minor criteria include a preceding respiratory or gastrointestinal infection. Laboratory data reveal an ESR > 20 mm/hr, polymorphonuclear cells ≥ 70%; and a leukocytosis > 8000/μl. Lastly, the syndrome responds to systemic steroids, not antibiotics. Potassium iodine has been used therapeutically with good results.

Cellulitis and leukocytoclastic vasculitis are the two diseases most commonly confused with Sweet's syndrome. In the present patient, the lack of response to a first-generation oral cephalosporin argues against cellulitis. Furthermore, there was no evidence of lymphangitis. Leukocytoclastic vasculitis can be excluded only by biopsy. If Sweet's syndrome is diagnosed, then a search should be made for an underlying malignancy.

The present patient was diagnosed with Sweet's syndrome based on her clinical symptoms, history of diabetes mellitus, and lack of response to cefalexin. A biopsy excluded leukocytoclastic vasculitis. She was treated with prednisone, and her skin condition resolved after 3 weeks of therapy.

Clinical Pearls

1. Sweet's syndrome should be considered when a patient presents with multiple areas of localized cellulitis or pustules that are not responding to antibiotic therapy.

2. Neutrophilic infiltration of the dermis, without associated leukocytoclastic vasculitis, is characteristic of Sweet's syndrome.

3. Sweet's syndrome often is associated with malignancies, especially acute myelogenous leukemia.

4. Sweet's syndrome is associated with leukocytosis, a polymorphonuclear cell predominance with a left shift, and an elevated ESR.

5. Treatment of Sweet's syndrome is with steroids or potassium iodine.

REFERENCES

1. Dompmartin A, Troussard X, Lorier E, et al: Sweet's syndrome associated with acute myelogenous leukemia: Atypical form simulating facial erysipelas. Int J Dermatol 1991; 30:644–647.
2. Park JW, Mehrotra B, Barnett BO, et al: The Sweet syndrome during therapy with granulocyte colony-stimulating factor. Ann Int Med 1992; 116:996–998.
3. Su WP, Fett DL, Gibson LE, Pittelkow MR: Sweet's syndrome: Acute febrile neutrophilic dermatosis. Semin Dermatol 1995; 14:173–178.

PATIENT 58

A 48-year-old man with fever and myalgias

A 48-year-old businessman who has been vacationing on eastern Long Island with his family suffers from an acute febrile illness with severe headache and myalgias 2 weeks after returning to Philadelphia. His symptoms gradually progress until he seeks medical attention. The patient denies cough, diarrhea, chest pain, night sweats, and rashes. He is allergic to penicillin, and he has a history of hypertension for which he is taking a beta-blocker and a diuretic. His temperature record has a dual-peak pattern (see figure).

Physical Examination: Temperature: 102°; pulse 118; respirations 14; blood pressure 200/94. General: relatively sick appearance. HEENT: no abnormalities. Chest: left lower lobe rales. Cardiac: left-sided S_4; grade I/VI systolic ejection murmur heard best at the base. Abdomen: questionable splenomegaly, soft, nontender, normal bowel sounds. Extremities: no rashes, edema, or clubbing.

Laboratory Findings: WBC 4100/μl with a left shift, 2% eosinophils, 3% atypical lymphocytes; platelets 75,000/μl. ESR 44 mm/hr. Hemoglobin and hematocrit: normal. BUN and creatinine: unremarkable. Aspartate aminotransferase: 1.5× normal. Alkaline phosphatase, creatine phosphokinase, serum electrolytes: normal. Electrocardiogram: inverted T waves in all leads. Chest radiograph: negative. Blood cultures: negative. Urinalysis: 2+ proteins, 1+ ketones.

Questions: What diagnosis is most probable? How would you proceed?

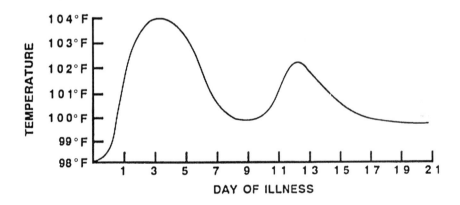

Diagnosis: Ehrlichiosis

Discussion: Ehrlichiosis is a rickettsial illness that resembles Rocky Mountain spotted fever, but usually presents without a rash. Two species of *Ehrlichia* are known at the present time: *E. equi* and *E. chaffeensis. E. equi* usually is referred to as human granulocytic ehrlichiosis (HGE) and is found predominantly in the northeast United States and around the Great Lakes in Michigan. It is transmitted by the deer tick *Ixodes scapularis,* which is the same tick that transmits Lyme disease and babesiosis. *E. chaffeensis* is responsible for human monocytic ehrlichiosis (HME).

HGE and HME present clinically in precisely the same fashion—the only difference is in the serologic results. Morulas, which are inclusionlike clusters of ehrlichiae in host cell vacuoles, are found in HGE infections but not *E. chaffeensis* infections. Morulas are found in monocytes in HME in about 30–40% of cases and are especially common in monocytes recovered from bone marrow biopsies.

Clinically, the two types of *Ehrlichia* are indistinguishable from each other and are hard to differentiate from Rocky Mountain spotted fever. In fact, if a patient has **Rocky Mountain spotted fever without a rash**, the physician should consider ehrlichiosis as a diagnostic possibility. *E. chaffeensis* (HME) has been associated with a variety of tick vectors (e.g., *Dermacentor variabilis, Ancylostoma, Emblyoma americanus,* heart dog tick) depending on the region of the country involved. As with Rocky Mountain spotted fever, a variety of nonspecific lab abnormalities occur, including thrombocytopenia, leukopenia, and mild elevations of transaminase. As with malaria, atypical lymphocytes usually are noted, although they may be at normal levels. In contrast to Rocky Mountain spotted fever, **edema on the dorsum of the hands and periorbital edema are *not* features of ehrlichiosis**, and these may be important differential points. Both Rocky Mountain spotted fever and ehrlichiosis have been associated with conjunctival suffusion.

The present patient was diagnosed with ehrlichiosis serologically. He was treated with doxycycline for 2 weeks, and all symptoms resolved.

Clinical Pearls

1. "Spotless" Rocky Mountain spotted fever suggests the diagnosis of ehrlichiosis.

2. Frequently, because the Ixodes tick carries ehrlichiosis as well as Lyme disease and babesiosis, Lyme disease tests are false positive in patients with ehrlichiosis.

3. Morulas are nearly always present in *E. equi* infections and are an important diagnostic clue. Morulas are seen less frequently, in monocytes, in patients with HME.

4. Atypical lymphocytes are seen in patients with ehrlichiosis, as are the mild elevations of serum transaminases also found in Rocky Mountain spotted fever.

REFERENCES
1. Dumler JS, Bakken JS: Ehrlichial diseases of humans: Emerging tick-borne infections. Clin Infect Dis 1995; 20:1102–1110.
2. Walker DH, Dumler JS: Emergence of the ehrlichioses as human health problems. Emerging Infect Dis 1996; 2:18–29.
3. Glushko GM: Human ehrlichiosis. Postgrad Med 1997; 101:225–230.

PATIENT 59

A 38-year-old man with fever, headache, and chills

A 38-year-old airline pilot presents to the emergency department with fever, headache, and chills 10 days after a trip to East Africa. The patient states that he developed some nonspecific, mild abdominal pain and diarrhea during the past week. He has been in good health and passed his annual pilot's physical exam. He denies cough, chest pain, rash, and night sweats. The patient has no known allergies, but has a history of gout.

Physical Examination: Temperature 39.2°; pulse 118; respirations 14; blood pressure 192/82. General: well appearing. HEENT: no abnormalities. Cardiac: unremarkable. Abdomen: normal bowel sounds, soft, nontender, no hepatosplenomegaly. Extremities: no edema or rashes.

Laboratory Findings: Hct 22%; WBC 4900/μl, no left shift; platelets 90,000/μl. Hemoglobin: 10 g/dl. Alkaline phosphatase: normal. Aspartate aminotransferase: 1.5× normal. Total bilirubin: slightly elevated. Urinalysis: 2+ protein, positive urobilinogen, 1+ bilirubin. Chest radiograph: no opacities or cardiomegaly. Blood and stool cultures: negative. Smear analysis: pending.

Question: What is the most likely diagnosis?

Diagnosis: Malaria

Discussion: Malaria, the most important protozoal infection in the world, is caused by four species of *Plasmodium*: *P. vivax, P. ovale, P. malariae,* and *P. falciparum.* The infectious form of the parasite, the sporozoid, is inoculated into the host by the mosquito. *P. falciparum* is potentially the most lethal of the species of malaria due to its higher levels of parasitemia affecting erythrocytes of all ages. Malaria is concentrated in Africa, Latin America, the Caribbean, and Asia. *P. vivax* is the usual species in Central America, whereas in Latin America *P. vivax* and *P. falciparum* are the usual pathogens. *P. ovale* is found primarily in Africa, where *P. vivax* is rare. *P. falciparum* is found predominantly in Africa, Haiti, and the islands of the western Pacific.

The signs and symptoms of malaria vary according to the stage of the infection. Symptoms can be highly variable, especially in the early phases, and it may be difficult to relate the symptoms to the illness. Fever is the most common sign. Patients also commonly complain of **chills, myalgias, arthralgias, headache, abdominal pain, and diarrhea**. Physical examination typically is unrevealing. Characteristic malarial paroxysms do not occur until the infection is well established, so that temperature curve analysis is not helpful in the initial stages of malarial infections. Physical examination may reveal splenomegaly in an established case.

Laboratory findings include **leukopenia, anemia, and thrombocytopenia**. *P. falciparum* causes the most prominent laboratory abnormalities. Hyponatremia in a patient with malaria suggests *P. falciparum* as the cause. Diagnosis of malaria is made by serial thick and thin smears every 6–12 hours over a 2-day period. Malarial smears should be obtained whenever a patient returning from a malarious area is febrile. There are a variety of nonspecific laboratory findings commonly seen in malaria, such as an **increase in the serum transaminases and bilirubin**.

The appropriate therapy for a patient with malaria depends upon whether the patient has chloroquine-resistant *P. falciparum* or *P. vivax*. Formerly, chloroquine resistance was a problem only with respect to *P. falciparum* infections; however chloroquine-resistant *P. vivax* has been reported in Indonesia, New Guinea, and Sumatra. When chloroquine-resistant *P. falciparum* cannot be excluded from the diagnosis, a combination of quinine and pyrimethamine combined with pyrimethamine sulfadoxine should be administered for 3 days. Doxycycline also may be used in combination with pyrimethamine sulfadoxine or quinine for 7 days. Chloroquine is still the mainstay of treatment for non-*P. falciparum* malaria.

In the present patient, headache, chills, and fever after a trip to East Africa were suspicious for malaria. Increased bilirubin also was indicative, and the diagnosis was confirmed when *P. falciparum* was identified on smear analysis (see figure). The patient received doxycycline therapy for 1 week because he was unable to tolerate other antimalarial medications, and he achieved a full recovery.

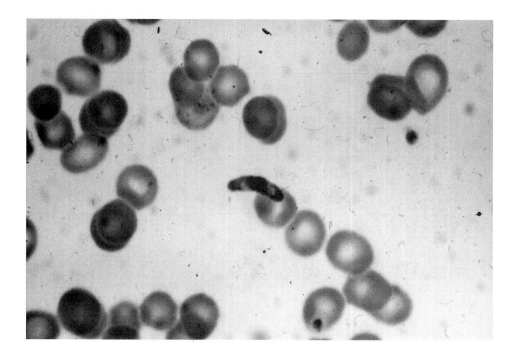

Clinical Pearls

1. Patients with malaria present with a nonspecific febrile illness in which headache and chills are the predominant clinical findings.

2. Splenomegaly occurs only after established infection.

3. Malaria must be differentiated from typhoid fever, which it resembles very closely in terms of clinical presentation and laboratory findings. Malaria is more likely in the presence of increased total bilirubin, thrombocytopenia, and atypical lymphocytes in the peripheral blood smear.

4. Non-*P. falciparum* malaria is treated with chloroquine (*P. malariae*) or chloroquine plus primaquine (*P. vivax* or *P. ovale*).

5. *P. falciparum* malaria with over 5% parasitemia is treated with quinine. Uncomplicated infections with less than 5% parasitemia may be treated with fansidar, mefloquine, or doxycycline.

REFERENCES

1. Krogstad DJ: Malaria as a re-emerging disease. Epidemiol Rev 1996; 18:77–89.
2. Murphy GS, Oldfield EC III: Falciparum malaria. Infect Dis Clin North Am 1996; 10:747–775.
3. Campbell CC: Malaria: An emerging and re-emerging global plague. FEMS Immunol Med Microbiol 1997; 18:325–331.
4. Stanley J: Malaria. Emerg Med Clin North Am 1997; 15:113–155.

PATIENT 60

A 26-year-old man with jaundice and renal failure

A 26-year-old man becomes sick 1 week after returning home from a hunting trip in the southeastern United States. His illness begins with headache, fever, and malaise. Subsequently, he complains of right upper quadrant abdominal pain. He denies cough, chest pain, night sweats, and diarrhea. His past medical history is significant for gout and congenital artery disease. He has no known allergies.

Physical Examination: Temperature 39.2°; pulse 112; respirations 18; blood pressure 130/70. HEENT: conjunctival suffusion (see figure). Cardiac: unremarkable. Abdomen: right upper quadrant tenderness, no organomegaly. Extremities: no rash or edema.

Laboratory Findings: WBC 12,800/μl with 87% neutrophils, 5% bands, 8% lymphocytes. Creatinine 2.1 mg/dl, BUN 18 mg/dl. Urinalysis: WBC 20/hpf, RBC 0/hpf, 2+ protein. Aspartate aminotransferase: 2× normal. Chest radiograph: minimal bilateral, linear lower lobe opacities; no pleural effusion.

Questions: What is your diagnosis? How would you pursue it?

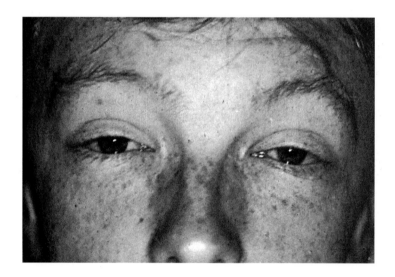

Diagnosis: Leptospirosis

Discussion: The combination of liver and renal involvement in an acutely ill, febrile patient who has been hunting in a rural setting suggests the diagnosis of leptospirosis. Preliminary findings typically are not prominent, as would be expected in hantavirus infection; leptospirosis frequently is subclinical. The infection is most commonly acquired by contact with aerosolized water that has been contaminated by animal urine containing leptospires. Jaundice develops in less than 10%. Patients tend to be veterinarians, campers, forest workers, or hunters.

The illness develops after an incubation period of 1–2 weeks, lasts approximately 1 week, and represents the septicemic phase of leptospirosis. The second, or immune, phase is characterized by **aseptic meningitis, rash, and occasionally uveitis**. In Weil's syndrome, the septicemic and immune phases occur together, and complications include jaundice, renal failure, hemorrhage, and myocarditis.

An important physical finding is **conjunctival suffusion** in a patient with elevated transaminases. Muscle tenderness and headaches are prominent. **Muscles are especially tender in the calf, back, abdomen, and neck areas**. Nearly all patients with leptospirosis develop some degree of nausea, vomiting, and abdominal pain. Headaches occurring a week or more after the onset of symptoms suggest aseptic meningitis.

Laboratory clues are important in differentiating leptospirosis from viral hepatitis. In viral hepatitis there is some degree of leukopenia in contrast to the **leukocytosis of leptospirosis**. Atypical lymphocytes usually are present (though numbers may be low) in viral hepatitis, but are conspicuous by their absence in leptospirosis. Renal abnormalities are not a feature of viral hepatitis.

The diagnosis of leptospirosis is made by isolating the leptospires from the blood or cerebrospinal fluid in the septicemic phase and from the urine during the immune phase. A presumptive diagnosis of leptospirosis can be made in a patient with a compatible illness on the finding of a microscopic agglutinin titer of $\geq 1:100$. Agglutinins appear after about 2 weeks and peak at 4–6 weeks.

The preferred treatment for leptospirosis is doxycycline. Beta lactams and chloramphenicol antibiotics are variably effective. Antibiotic therapy may delay or abort the antibody response, and cross-reactions can occur with other spirochetal organisms.

The present patient exhibited an acute febrile illness characterized by fever, headache, myalgias, and jaundice. Leptospires were isolated from his blood, and he was treated with doxycycline for 2 weeks. His recovery was uneventful.

Clinical Pearls

1. "Viral hepatitis" with leukocytosis, no atypical lymphocytes, and renal abnormalities suggests the diagnosis of leptospirosis.

2. Anicteric hepatitis is the most common clinical manifestation of leptospirosis. Weil's syndrome, of which jaundice is a feature, occurs in less than 10% of patients.

REFERENCES

1. Farr RW: Leptospirosis. Clin Infect Dis 1995; 21:1–6.
2. Vinetz JM, Glass GE, Flexner CE, et al: Sporadic urban leptospirosis. Ann Intern Med 1996; 125:794–798.
3. Dupont H, Dupont-Perdrizet D, Perie JL, et al: Leptospirosis: Prognostic factors associated with mortality. Clin Infect Dis 1997; 25:720–724.

PATIENT 61

A 19-year-old woman with rash and sore throat

A 19-year-old college student presents with a 1-week history of fever, malaise, and sore throat. She reports puffiness of her upper eyelids and a rash over her entire body, including her palms and soles. The school health service diagnosed streptococcal pharyngitis 4 days ago, on the basis of a rapid strep test. The patient denies contact with other students with strep throat. She has no pets aside from tropical fish. She denies cough, chest pain, headache, abdominal pain, and diarrhea. Past medical history is significant only for endometriosis, and she has no known allergies.

Physical Examination: Temperature 38.8°; pulse 72; respirations 18; blood pressure 110/50. General: tired, but well appearing. HEENT: bilateral upper eyelid edema; exudative pharyngitis with palatal petechiae; bilateral posterior cervical adenopathy. Cardiac: unremarkable. Abdomen: soft, nontender, no splenomegaly, liver not enlarged. Extremities: normal.

Laboratory Findings: WBC 6400/μl with 59% neutrophils, 25% lymphocytes, 10% atypical lymphocytes, 6% monocytes; platelets normal; ESR 66 mm/hr. BUN and creatinine: normal. Aspartate aminotransferase: 2× normal. Alkaline phosphatase: normal. Monospot test: negative. Rapid strep test: positive. Gram stain of throat: negative for polymorphonuclear cells. Antistreptolysin O: 110.

Question: What is the probable diagnosis given this patient's presentation?

Diagnosis: Infectious mononucleosis caused by Epstein-Barr virus

Discussion: Infectious mononucleosis is caused by a variety of agents (e.g., cytomegalovirus, toxoplasmosis) but is most commonly due to Epstein-Barr virus (EBV). EBV infectious mononucleosis typically affects young adults, although it may occur in all age groups. Patients usually present with progressive malaise, fatigue, fever, and sore throat. The disease runs the spectrum from minimal illness to life-threatening disease. The diagnosis of EBV infectious mononucleosis is based on clinical, hematologic, and serologic criteria. Clinical features include fever, sore throat, and adenopathy. Hematologic characteristics include ≥ 50% lymphocytes and ≥ 10% atypical lymphocytes. Serologic criteria include the presence of heterophile antibodies (a positive monospot test) and permanent antibody response to EBV.

The differential diagnosis generally includes streptococcal pharyngitis. Note that the presence of group A streptococci does not establish the diagnosis of streptococcal pharyngitis; 30% of patients with EBV infectious mononucleosis have concomitant streptococcal colonization of the pharynx. Moreover, a positive throat culture for group A streptococci does not differentiate colonization from infection. It is important to make this differentiation because there is a high incidence of drug reaction in EBV infectious mononucleosis, and a patient with group A streptococcal colonization should not be treated.

Early findings in EBV infectious mononucleosis include bilateral upper eyelid edema and a maculopapular rash. Splenomegaly does not usually occur until the second or third week of illness; thus, the absence of splenomegaly early in the disease does not argue against the diagnosis. The rash and eye findings are found later in the illness, and the monospot test positivity increases over time. A negative monospot test early in the illness (as in the present patient) does not rule out EBV infectious mononucleosis. The monospot test should be obtained weekly (up to 6 weeks) until positive.

A complete blood cell count with a predominance of lymphocytes suggests viral rather than bacterial characteristics. The presence of atypical lymphocytes also strongly argues against group A streptococcal pharyngitis. In addition, the ESR is increased in EBV infectious mononucleosis, but is not a factor in group A streptococcal pharyngitis. Similarly, serum transaminases increase early in EBV infectious mononucleosis, but do not increase in streptococcal pharyngitis. Anterior cervical adenopathy, which is associated with Group A streptococcal pharyngitis, is a common specific finding in a wide variety of infectious diseases involving the oral pharynx. However, bilateral posterior cervical adenopathy suggests a systemic disease and strongly favors the diagnosis of EBV infectious mononucleosis.

Patient recovery typically is uneventful over several weeks. Complications include airway compromise due to enlarged tonsils, autoimmune hemolytica anemia, central nervous system involvement, and splenic rupture. Steroids are useful when complications arise. All patients with EBV infectious mononucleosis should be advised against engaging in physical activity for at least 1 month following clinical onset of illness.

The present patient did not improve with oral penicillin therapy, suggesting that she had streptococcal colonization rather than true infection. The clinical finding of posterior cervical adenopathy also supported the diagnosis of nonstreptococcal pharyngitis. The antistreptolysin titer was not increased, which argued against the diagnosis of streptococcal pharyngitis, but the test was performed early in the illness—there may not have been time for an increase. The Gram stain of the throat showed no polymorphonuclear cell reaction in a patient with a positive throat culture for group A streptococcal pharyngitis. The patient became monospot-positive after 10 weeks. She recovered slowly, but completely.

Clinical Pearls

1. Exudative pharyngitis with posterior cervical adenopathy in a young adult should be considered EBV infectious mononucleosis until proven otherwise.

2. Streptococcal colonization is common in EBV infectious mononucleosis as well as in other causes of viral pharyngitis and should *not* be treated.

3. An increased ESR and increased serum transaminases in a patient with pharyngitis favors the diagnosis of EBV infectious mononucleosis.

4. Over 20% atypical lymphocytes in the peripheral smear points to EBV infectious mononucleosis, but also may be seen in cytomegalovirus infectious mononucleosis.

REFERENCES

1. Khanna R, Burrows SR, Moss DJ: Immune regulation of Epstein-Barr virus-associated diseases. Microbiol Rev 1995; 59:387–405.
2. Niedobitek G, Agathanggelou A, Herbst H, et al: Epstein-Barr virus (EBV) infection in infectious mononucleosis: Virus latency, replication and phenotype of EBV-infected cells. J Pathol 1997; 182:151–159.
3. Ternak G, Szucs G, Uj M: The serological signs of Epstein-Barr virus activity in the elderly. Acta Microbiol Immunol Hung 1997; 44:133–140.

PATIENT 62

A 20-year-old man with nonproductive cough and low-grade fevers

A 20-year-old college student presents with a 3-week history of nonproductive cough, myalgia, and low-grade fevers, recently followed by right ear pain. He had "pneumonia" during his senior year of high school, which cleared with antibiotic therapy, but otherwise has been in good health. He has no risk factors for human immunodeficiency virus and denies headache, chills, and chest or abdominal pain. Past medical history is significant for Osgood-Schlatter disease as a child.

Physical Examination: Temperature 38°; pulse 70; respirations 16; blood pressure 122/74. General: well appearing. HEENT: mild erythema in oropharynx, some ear tenderness. Chest: right lower lobe rales. Cardiac: normal S_1S_2 with a grade I/VI ejection murmur at the base. Abdomen: soft, nontender, no hepatosplenomegaly. Extremities: concentric, red, nontender, and nonblanching lesions more than 2 cm in diameter on arms and legs.

Laboratory Findings: WBC 9900/μl, no left shift. Creatinine and BUN: normal. Cold agglutinin titer: positive at 1:128. Serum transaminase and alkaline phosphatase: normal. Urinalysis: unremarkable. Chest radiograph: nonspecific right lower lobe opacity; no hilar adenopathy or pleural effusions (see figure).

Question: What is the most likely clinical diagnosis?

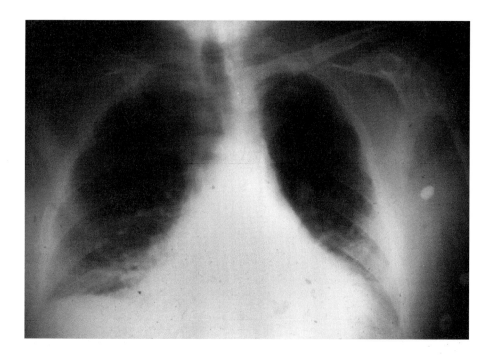

Diagnosis: *Mycoplasma pneumoniae* pneumonia

Discussion: Mycoplasma pneumonia is primarily a disease of young adults. It frequently presents with a nonproductive cough that persists over days or weeks. Temperatures almost always are less than 38.8° and often are accompanied by mild headache and/or myalgia.

The key to the diagnosis of Mycoplasma pneumonia and other atypical pneumonias is extrapulmonary findings. Common symptoms are loose stools/diarrhea, ear involvement (e.g., bullous myringitis, otitis media), and a mild, nonexudative pharyngitis. Extrapulmonary manifestations of *Mycoplasma pneumoniae* infection, e.g., Erythema multiforme, should be regarded as indications of systemic infectious disease.

Laboratory tests are unhelpful in the diagnosis, except for the cold agglutinin titer, which may show a transient increase. The higher the cold agglutinin titer is above 1:64, the more likely the cause is *M. pneumoniae*. *M. pneumoniae* may be cultured from respiratory secretions or diagnosed serologically.

Note that unlike legionnaires' disease, mycoplasmal pneumonia does not ordinarily involve the liver. Moreover, legionnaires' disease is not associated with pharyngitis or ear involvement. The presence of cold agglutinins also argues strongly against the diagnosis of legionnaires' disease.

Mycoplasma pneumonia is treated with doxycycline or a macrolide for 2 weeks. β-lactam antibiotics are ineffective. Treatment with second-generation tetracyclines decreases the excretion time of the organism in the sputum. Antimicrobial therapy generally has no effect on the clinical illness or laboratory findings, but improves the patient's feeling of well being. Importantly, antimicrobial therapy has no effect on the nonproductive cough characteristic of Mycoplasma pneumonia.

The present patient's low-grade fever, nonproductive cough, and highly elevated cold agglutinin titer suggested the diagnosis of Mycoplasma pneumonia. His *Mycoplasma* IgM titer subsequently was positive. He made an uneventful recovery after 2 weeks of doxycycline therapy.

Clinical Pearls

1. Community-acquired pneumonia and ear pain or sore throat suggest the diagnosis of Mycoplasma pneumonia.

2. Loose stools/diarrhea but no abdominal pain in a patient with community-acquired pneumonia suggests *Mycoplasma* or *Legionella* infection.

3. Erythema multiforme in a nonmedicated patient with community-acquired pneumonia points to the diagnosis of Mycoplasma pneumonia.

4. Relative bradycardia and increased serum transaminases are *not* features of Mycoplasma pneumonia.

5. The higher the cold agglutinin is above 1:64 in a patient with a nonproductive cough and community-acquired pneumonia, the more likely the diagnosis is Mycoplasma pneumonia.

6. Consolidation and noticeable pleural effusions on chest radiograph are not features of Mycoplasma pneumonia.

REFERENCES
1. Cunha BA, Johnson DH: Mycoplasma pneumonia. Emerg Med 1997;29:112–114.
2. Leong MA, Nachajon R, Ruchelli E, Allen JL: Bronchitis obliterans due to Mycoplasma pneumonia. 1997;23:375–381.

PATIENT 63

A 19-year-old woman with fever, cough, and sore throat

A 19-year-old college student presents with fever, cough, and sore throat of 4-week duration. The student health service prescribed erythromycin, and she took the antibiotic faithfully despite nausea and diarrhea, but the low-grade fevers and nonproductive cough persisted. One week after the onset of illness, persistent hoarseness developed. The patient denies headaches, abdominal pain, weight loss, and night sweats, and she has no known allergies. Her past medical history includes an appendectomy.

Physical Examination: Temperature 38.6°; pulse 78; respirations 22; blood pressure 120/60. General: well appearing, but coughing. HEENT: some pharyngeal edema, otherwise normal. Chest: minimal right lower lobe rales. Cardiac: normal. Abdomen: soft, nontender, no organomegaly.

Laboratory Findings: WBC 8900/μl; ESR 32 mm/hr. Liver function tests: normal. BUN and creatinine: unremarkable. Urinalysis: 1+ protein. Cold agglutinin titer 1:4. Electrocardiogram: normal. Chest radiograph: right lower lung opacity (see figure).

Question: What diagnosis is suggested by the patient's clinical presentation?

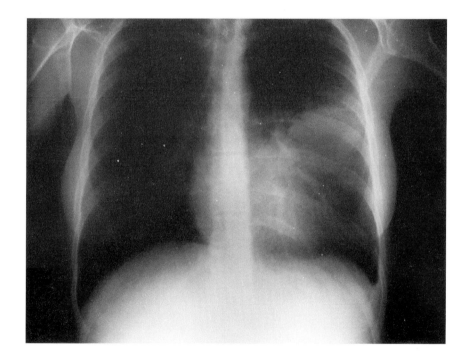

Diagnosis: *Chlamydia pneumoniae* pneumonia

Discussion: Chlamydia pneumonia is one of the most common atypical pneumonias in young adults; the other is Mycoplasma pneumonia. Patients present with illness resembling Mycoplasma pneumonia, but hoarseness also is a feature. Clues to the diagnosis of Chlamydia pneumonia are a lack of response to erythromycin, which is universally effective with mycoplasmosis, and less frequent incidence of diarrhea. Routine lab tests are generally unhelpful. Cold agglutinins are not elevated in contrast to the scenario in patients infected by *Mycoplasma pneumoniae*. Finally, chest radiographic findings are similar in both disorders, featuring wispy lower lung opacities without consolidation or effusion. Pneumonia caused by *Chlamydia pneumoniae* has been associated with coronary artery disease and asthma.

Chlamydia pneumonia may be diagnosed clinically if a patient with Mycoplasma-like illness and laryngitis responds to doxycycline after failing to improve on erythromycin therapy. A definitive diagnosis can be made by obtaining specific IgM *C. pneumoniae* titers. *C. pneumoniae* antibody immunoglobulin G titers indicate past exposure but are not helpful in making the diagnosis of acute infection. The treatment of Chlamydia pneumonia is doxycycline, with macrolides as alternative agents.

The present patient was treated with doxycycline for 2 weeks. Her *C. pneumoniae* IgM titers were highly elevated. The hoarseness resolved in 3 days, and she returned to her college after completion of therapy.

Clinical Pearls

1. The diagnosis of Chlamydia pneumonia should be suspected in a patient with mononucleosis-like illness unresponsive to erythromycin.

2. Disorder resembling Mycoplasma pneumonia but with hoarseness and/or laryngitis is considered Chlamydia pneumonia until proven otherwise.

3. Doxycycline rather than erythromycin is the drug of choice for Chlamydia pneumonia.

4. Specific IgM *Chlamydia* titers confirm the diagnosis. Nonspecific *Chlamydia* titers are not helpful and should not be obtained.

REFERENCES
1. Kuo CC, Jackson LA, Campbell LA, et al: *Chlamydia pneumoniae*. Clin Microbiol Rev 1995; 8:451–461.
2. Cunha BA, Ortega AM: Atypical pneumonias. Postgrad Med 1996; 99:123–132.
3. Cunha BA: Atypical pathogens are important in community-acquired pneumonias. Controversies in Pulmonary Medicine. 1998; 2:2–15.

PATIENT 64

A 50-year-old man with cough and fever

A 50-year-old man is admitted to the hospital with a 2-week history of fever and cough. A chest radiograph obtained in his physician's office 1 week prior to admission revealed an indistinct opacity in the right lower lobe. His physician prescribed an oral cephalosporin, which the patient took faithfully until admission, but he worsened while on the antibiotic. He complains of headache, mental confusion, and 3 days of diarrhea over the previous week. The patient denies night sweats and weight loss, and his appetite is good. His past medical history is significant for rheumatoid arthritis and hypertension. He has no known allergies.

Physical Examination: Temperature 104°; pulse 96; respirations 24; blood pressure 190/88. General: ill appearing. HEENT: normal. Chest: rales at the right base and left apex. Cardiac: unremarkable except grade II/VI systolic ejection murmur at apex. Abdomen: soft, nontender, no organomegaly. Extremities: no edema or rash.

Laboratory Findings: WBC 28,200/μl. Creatinine 2.4 mg/dl, BUN 36 mg/dl. Urinalysis: 2+ protein, RBC 4/hpf, WBC 0/hpf. Serum electrolyes: normal except for Na$^+$ 116 mEq/L. Serum phosphorus: decreased. Liver function tests: increased. Aspartate aminotransferase: 1.5× normal. Alkaline phosphatase: normal. Chest radiograph: right lower lobe, left upper lobe, and lingular opacities; no cavitation or effusion.

Question: What disorder is suggested by the patient's symptoms and course (see figure)?

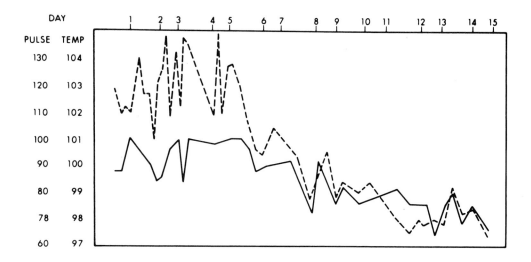

Diagnosis: Legionnaires' disease

Discussion: Of the *Legionella* species, *L. pneumophila* remains the most common cause of legionnaires' disease. Legionnaires' disease occurs mainly in the elderly during late summer and early fall, but may be seen in all age groups year round. Outbreaks have been associated with contaminated water, ice, hot tubs, showers, and excavations.

Patients with legionnaires' disease have a rapidly progressive community-acquired pneumonia (CAP) with extrapulmonary features. Extrapulmonary features that suggest legionnaires' disease in a patient with CAP include mental confusion, headaches, abdominal pain, and diarrhea. While infection with *Mycoplasma pneumoniae* frequently is accompanied by diarrhea, central nervous system and abdominal findings usually are not a feature. Patients with legionnaires' disease may have a productive or nonproductive cough and rapidly progressive, asymmetrical opacities on chest radiograph. Blood cultures are negative, and sputum does not contain a predominant organism.

Legionnaires' disease is suggested by a constellation of lab findings, including abnormal liver function tests with or without hypophosphatemia and hyponatremia. A key physical finding is relative bradycardia (pulse-temperature deficit). The usual pathogens causing CAP are not associated with relative bradycardia. Therefore, relative bradycardia in a patient with CAP who is not on β-blockers strongly suggests atypical pneumonia due to legionnaires' disease, psittacosis, or Q fever. It should be noted, however, that hospitalized patients with CAP have similar manifestations whether they have infection with "typical" or "atypical" pathogens.

The clinical diagnosis of legionnaires' disease is based on the association of extrapulmonary findings, abnormal liver function tests, and relative bradycardia with nosocomial or CAP. The diagnosis is confirmed by obtaining a legionellae serology immediately and 6 weeks later. Antibiotic treatment may blunt or abolish the antibody response. If the patient is bringing up sputum, then direct fluorescent antibody of the sputum for legionellae may provide an immediate diagnosis. Antigens for legionellae present early in the illness; thus, a negative titer does not rule out the diagnosis.

Beta lactam antibiotics, typically used for community-acquired pneumonia, are ineffective in legionnaire's disease. Doxycycline is effective treatment for all *Legionella* species. Erythromycin also can be used; however, it costs twice as much as doxycycline and may cause or exacerbate diarrhea and phlebitis. Furthermore, there have been several reports of erythromycin failures in the treatment of legionnaires' disease. Quinolones, particularly levofloxacin, and azithromycin also are effective in legionnaires' disease. Rifampin has been used to potentiate the limited anti-*Legionella* activity of erythromycin, but is not necessary with doxyciline, azithromycin, or quinolones. Doxycycline is prescribed in high doses for the first 72 hours (200 mg IV q12h) and then decreased to the usual dose (100 mg IV or PO q 12h) to complete a 2–4 week regimen.

In the present patient, extrapulmonary findings suggested not only atypical pneumonia, but specifically legionnaires' disease. The patient was started on intravenous doxycycline therapy, with slow response over the first week and improvement the second week. Recovery was achieved in 3 weeks.

Clinical Pearls

1. Diarrhea in a patient with CAP suggests legionnaires' disease or mycoplasmal pneumonia.

2. Rapidly progressive, asymmetrical opacities are characteristic of legionnaires' disease, but no appearance on chest radiograph is pathognomonic.

3. Relative bradycardia or an unexplained increase in serum transaminases in a patient with CAP points to legionnaires' disease, psittacosis, or Q fever.

4. Extrapulmonary features in CAP are the most important factor in identifying atypical pneumonia.

REFERENCES
1. Cunha BA: The diagnostic significance of fever curves. Infect Dis Clin North Am 1996; 10:33–44.
2. Cunha BA: Severe community-acquired pneumonia. J Crit Illness 1997; 12:711–721.
3. Cunha BA: Clinial features of legionnaires' disease. Semin Respir Infect 1998; 13:116-127.
4. Edelstein PH: Antimicrobial chemotherapy for legionnaires' disease: Time for a change. Ann Intern Med 1998; 129:328.

PATIENT 65

A 76-year-old woman status post aortic valve replacement with fever

A 76-year-old woman underwent three-vessel coronary artery bypass grafting (CABG) and aortic valve replacement 7 months ago. She presents with a 38.8°C temperature of 3-day duration and generalized fatigue. Low-grade fevers have been present over the previous month. She denies cough, chest pain, headache, myalgias, night sweats, abdominal pain, and diarrhea. Previous medical history includes insulin-dependent diabetes mellitus and congestive heart failure. There are no known allergies to antibiotics.

Physical Examination: Temperature 39.4°; pulse 86; respirations 22; blood pressure 120/62. General: ill-appearing. HEENT: no abnormalities. Chest: decreased breath sounds at both bases. Cardiac: normal S_1S_2, grade II/IV systolic murmur at the apex. Abdomen: soft, nontender, no organomegaly. Extremities: bilateral pedal edema, no rashes.

Laboratory Findings: WBC 21,000/μl with 87% polymorphonuclear cells, 5% bands, 6% lymphocytes, 2% monocytes. Creatinine 2.4 mg/dl. Urinalysis: WBC 56/hpf, RBC 4/hpf, 2+ protein. Blood cultures: two sets obtained from different sites are growing gram-positive cocci in clusters that have not yet been identified (see figure). Chest radiograph: bilateral peripheral vascular congestion with small pleural effusions.

Question: What is the most likely cause of this patient's clinical presentation?

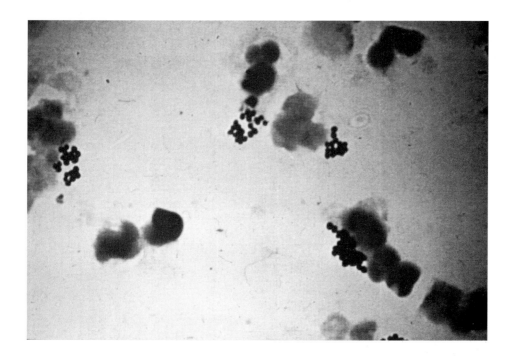

Diagnosis: Staphylococcal prosthetic valve endocarditis

Discussion: The overall incidence of prosthetic valve endocarditis (PVE) is 1–4%. Early PVE occurs from 60 days to 1 year after insertion of a mechanical or bioprosthetic valve. The most common bacterial organism involved is *Staphylococcus epidermidis* (25–30%) followed by *Staphylococcus aureus* (15–20%) and viridans streptococci (5–10%). Aerobic gram-negative bacilli fungi (especially *Candida* and *Aspergillus* species) and diphtheroids also are important causes of PVE. The diagnosis of PVE is made by positive blood cultures when other sources for bacteremia have been ruled out. Negative blood cultures may indicate infection with *Legionella,* mycobacteria, *Aspergillus,* or *Hemophilus* species in a symptomatic patient. Late PVE occurs 1 year after valve insertion and, similar to native valve endocarditis, the most commonly isolated organisms are the viridans streptococci. *S. epidermidis* is the second most likely pathogen in this setting.

Early PVE caused by *S. epidermidis* reflects perioperative valve contamination from direct wound inoculation, bypass pump contamination, or an infected intravascular catheter or pressure monitoring device. Valvular dysfunction is associated with dehiscence, valve ring abscess formation, leaflet destruction, and paravalvular leak. Extension of the abscess beyond the ring valve can cause myocardial abscess, septal perforation, and purulent pericarditis. Septic embolic events to the central nervous system and periphery can cause brain or deep tissue hemorrhagic infarcts, abscesses, and mycotic aneurysms.

Clinically, patients present with two or more of the following: fevers, a new or changing regurgitant murmur, petechiae, Osler nodes (rarely), Roth spots and Janeway lesions, splenomegaly and anemia (more common in late PVE), leukocytosis (more common in early PVE), normal or abnormal urinalysis, hematuria, and elevated creatinine secondary to glomerulonephritis. The most common clinical presentation is fever with focal deficits secondary to central nervous system emboli.

Transesophageal echocardiography (TEE) is more sensitive than transthoracic echocardiography (TTE) in detecting vegetations and valvular complications. A computed tomography scan of the head should be obtained for all patients with neurologic symptoms. If the scan is negative, but symptoms persist, a cerebral angiogram or MRI is obtained to rule out a cerebral mycotic aneurysm. Once a clinical diagnosis of PVE is made, the patient should empirically be started on vancomycin and genta-micin until blood culture results are finalized. Results can take up to 3 weeks because the mortality rate in PVE is as high as 30%. Once sensitivities are available, serum bactericidal levels of antibodies should be maintained. Repeat blood cultures should be obtained daily for the first few days and weekly thereafter until completion of therapy. Therapy is continued for 6 weeks after the last set of positive blood cultures. If infection is persistent and blood cultures remain positive after 2 weeks of therapy, consider occult abscess or mycotic aneurysm and the necessity of valve replacement.

Surgical intervention is indicated in the following situations: congestive heart failure with valve dysfunction, acute valve obstruction, fungal PVE (replace valve within 48–72 hours), persistent bacteremia with no other source after 2 weeks of therapy, relapse after appropriate therapy, one major or two or more embolic events, vegetations on TTE or TEE, heart block, ruptured ventricular septal defect, early PVE < 60 days, or paravalvular leak.

In the present patient, physical examination revealed fever but no localizing findings. Her blood cultures were all positive for *S. epidermidis*. She underwent reoperation and has been free of infection since her prosthetic valve was replaced.

Clinical Pearls

1. Late prosthetic valve endocarditis presents similarly to native valve endocarditis and is caused by the same kinds of organisms.

2. Bacteremia occurring in the setting of a prosthetic valve does not always indicate endocarditis.

3. Transesophageal echocardiography is more sensitive than transthoracic echocardiography in making the diagnosis of prosthetic valve endocarditis.

REFERENCES

1. Mansur AJ, Grinberg M, Lemosdaluz P: The complications of infective endocarditis. Arch Intern Med 1992; 152:2428–2432.
2. Whitener C, Caputo GM, Weitekamp MR, Karchmer AW: Endocarditis due to coagulase-negative staphylococci: Microbiologic, epidemiologic, and clinical considerations (review). Infect Dis Clin North Am 1993; 7:81–96.
3. David TE: The surgical treatment of patients with prosthetic valve endocarditis. Semin Thorac Cardiovasc Surg 1995; 7:47–53.
4. Threlkeld MG, Cobbs CG: Infectious disorders of prosthetic valves and intravascular devices. In Mandell GL, Douglas RG Jr, Bennett JE (eds): Principles and Practice of Infectious Diseases. New York, Churchill Livingstone, 1995, pp 783–793.
5. Stanbridge TN, Isalska BJ: Aspects of prosthetic valve endocarditis. J Infect 1997; 35:1–6.
6. Vlessis AA, Khaki A, Grunkemeier GL, et al: Risk, diagnosis and management of prosthetic valve endocarditis: A review. J Heart Valve Dis 1997; 6:443–465.

PATIENT 66

A 65-year-old woman with fever and fatigue

A 65-year-old woman presents in the summer with a 4-day history of fevers to 40°C, shaking chills, severe fatigue, and decreased oral intake. She reports that she removed a tick from her arm 1 month ago. She is a resident of eastern Long Island.

Physical Examination: Temperature 39.8°; pulse 86; respirations 20; blood pressure 120/70. HEENT: normal. Chest: clear to auscultation. Cardiac: normal S_1S_2, with a grade II/VI systolic ejection murmur. Abdomen: soft, nontender, no hepatosplenomegaly. Extremities: no edema or rashes. Neurologic: no focal deficits; lethargic but alert and oriented to person, place, and time.

Laboratory Findings: Hct 32%; WBC 8900/μl with 60% polymorphonuclear cells, 6% bands, 28% lymphocytes, 6% monocytes; platelets 72,000/μl; hemoglobin 10.8 mg/dl. Na^+ 130 mEq/L, K^+ 3.8 mEq/L, HCO_3^- 22 mEq/L, Cl^- 90 mEq/L. Glucose 120 mg/dl. Aspartate aminotransferase 134 IU/L, alanine aminotransferase 66 IU/L, alkaline phosphatase 120 IU/L. Lactate dehydrogenase 468 IU/L, total bilirubin 2 mg/dl. Giemsa stain of blood: see figure. Chest radiograph: no opacities.

Question: What is your diagnosis?

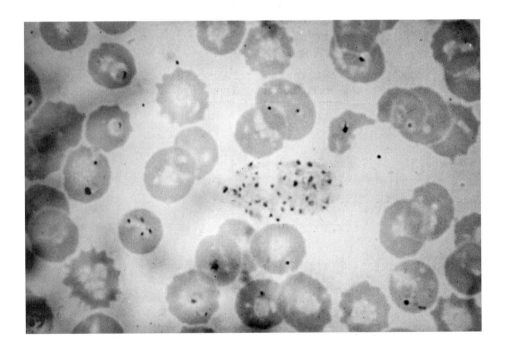

Diagnosis: Babesiosis

Discussion: Babesiosis is an intraerythrocytic zoonosis transmitted to humans by ticks or by blood transfusions. Transmission is mainly from bites by *Ixodes dammini* ticks, the principle vector of *Borrelia burgdorferi,* which is the agent for Lyme disease. Lyme disease can be transmitted concurrently. Other ixodid ticks that transmit disease include *I. scapularis, I. ricinus,* and *I. pacificus.* The white-footed mouse, *Peromycus leicopus,* is the principle reservoir for *Babesia microti,* the species that most commonly causes infection in the northeastern United States. In California, infection caused by *B. equi* also has been reported. *B. divergens,* which causes severe and sometimes fatal disease in splenectomized patients, and *B. bovis* have been reported mostly in Europe. WA1 is a new species recently identified in Washington State.

Human babesiosis is most common in the summer months, and most cases occur on Nantucket Island, Martha's Vineyard, Block Island, eastern Long Island, Shelter Island, and Fire Island, and in mainland Connecticut.

Patients can present with a mild, self-limited illness; malaria-like symptoms; or severe disease. The incubation period for tick-transmitted *B. microti* is 1–4 weeks, but most patients recall no tick bite. In transfusion-associated babesiosis, the incubation period is 6–9 weeks. Most patients complain of a gradual onset of malaise, fatigue, and anorexia, followed by high fever with chills and drenching night sweats, myalgia, and headache. Risk factors for severe illness include advanced age, underlying medical problems, an immunocompromised state, and Lyme disease in an endemic area. In Europe, the greatest risk factor is splenectomy, and most splenectomy-related cases are fatal.

Clinically, there may be hepatosplenomegaly with jaundice and hemolytic anemia, thrombocytopenia, and elevated serum bilirubin, alkaline phosphatase, aminotransferases, and lactate dehydrogenase. Lymphadenopathy is not a feature. Severe illness can result in hypotension, hemoglobulinemia, hemoglobinuria, renal failure, and death. A diagnosis of babesiosis should be entertained in any patient with a febrile illness in an endemic area (with or without a history of tick bite), clinical and serologic evidence of Lyme disease with unexplained anemia, or malaria-like symptoms with no risk factors for malaria.

Diagnosis of babesiosis is made by Wright or Giemsa-stained thick and thin peripheral blood smears. The organisms are seen as small intraerythrocytic ring forms with a tetrad of budding *Babesia* trophozoites. The "Maltese cross" sign is diagnostic. The absence of pigment deposits, schizonts, or gametocytes distinguishes babesiosis from *Plasmodium falciparum.* Indirect immunofluorescence antibody testing can also be used to make the diagnosis, with titers remaining elevated for several months after symptoms have resolved.

Most patients with *B. microti* recover with treatment. Therapy in symptomatic patients is a 7- to 10-day course of quinine sulfate and oral or intravenous clindamycin. In severe cases, or in a splenic patient with high levels of parasitemia or hemolysis, exchange transfusions in addition to quinine and clindamycin are recommended.

In the present patient, the diagnosis was confirmed by demonstrating the parasite in stained peripheral smears. The patient was treated with oral quinine and clindamycin, and she made a complete recovery.

Clinical Pearls

1. Most infections with *Babesia microti* are subclinical.

2. Patients who develop clinical illness are > 50 years old, and two thirds have intact spleens.

3. Twenty percent of babesiosis is transmitted concurrently with *Borrelia burgdorferi,* the agent that causes Lyme disease.

4. Suspect babesiosis in a patient with malaria-like illness who has not travelled recently in a malarious area.

REFERENCES

1. Spach DL, Liles WC, et al: Tickborne disease in the United States. N Engl J Med 1993; 329:936–947.
2. Pruthi RK, Marshall WF, Wiltsie JC, Persing DH: Human babesiosis. Mayo Clin Proc 1995; 70:853–862.
3. Boustani MR, Gelfand JA: Babesiosis. Clin Infect Dis 1996; 22:611–615.
4. Dao AH: Human babesiosis. Compr Ther 1996; 22:713–718.

PATIENT 67

**A 35-year-old man with acquired immunodeficiency syndrome
and watery diarrhea**

A 35-year-old man with a CD_4 count of $70/\mu l$ presents with a 2-month history of nausea, profuse and watery diarrhea, crampy abdominal pain, weight loss (totaling 20 pounds), chronic nonproductive cough, and generalized malaise. One month before admission he went on a hiking trip with friends, two of whom developed a diarrheal illness shortly afterwards but have since recovered. He was on trimethroprim-sulfamethoxazole as prophylaxis against pneumonia caused by *Pneumocystis carinii,* but stopped taking it because of worsening nausea.

Physical Examination: Temperature 37.5°; pulse 120; respirations 20; blood pressure 80/50. General: cachectic and dehydrated. Abdomen: diffuse tenderness, hyperactive bowel sounds. Chest: clear.

Laboratory Findings: Na^+ 128 mEq/L, K^+ 3.0 mEq/L. BUN 43 mg/dl, creatinine 2.0 mg/dl. Amylase 560 IU/L. Chest radiograph: clear. Abdominal radiograph: distended loops of small bowel. Gram stain of stool: see figure.

Questions: What diagnosis is most probable? How would you proceed?

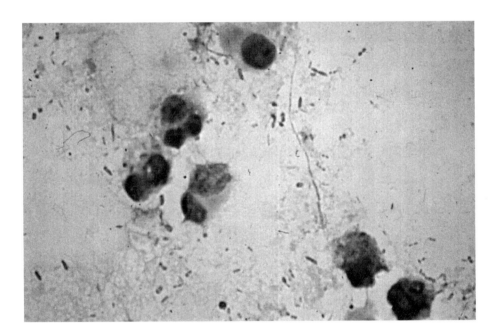

Diagnosis: Cryptosporidiosis

Discussion: Cryptosporidiosis is acquired after ingestion of less than 150 oocysts of the protozoan parasite, *Cryptosporidium parvum,* which is shed in the feces of infected animals or humans. *C. parvum* causes a self-limited gastroenteritis in normal hosts, but in the immunocompromised, infection can be chronic and even fatal. It is a ubiquitous, enteric pathogen that can infect the gastrointestinal tract from the pharynx to the colon, the biliary tree, and the respiratory tract. After ingestion, the oocysts excyst to release sporozoites that enter the mucosal cells of the gastrointestinal tract. When later expelled into the environment, oocysts can remain viable over a wide temperature range for many months.

Cysts are acquired from infected water supplies, e.g., artesian wells, untreated surface water, filtered public water supplies, and swimming pools. Waterborne epidemics have occurred because the organism is highly resistant to routine chlorination. Spread between homosexual and heterosexual partners has been reported. Nosocomial outbreaks have occurred in hospitals, household pets, and laboratory and farm animals. Children in day care centers and their household contacts are all susceptible.

After ingestion, symptoms develop within 1–2 weeks. Patients complain of diarrhea with or without crampy abdominal pain, low-grade fever, generalized malaise, fatigue, anorexia, nausea, and vomiting. The diarrhea may be intermittent and scant, or continuous. Immunocompromised patients have chronic, persistent, voluminous diarrhea with fluid losses of up to 25 liters a day due to autoreinfection as the sporozoites excyst within the gastrointestinal tract. These patients present with severe abdominal pain, weight loss and wasting, secretory diarrhea, malabsorption syndrome, and steatorrhea. The presence of right upper quadrant and midepigastric pain suggests pancreatitis, papillary stenosis, and biliary tract involvement with acalculous cystitis, sclerosing cholangitis, or hepatitis. Other clinical manifestations include reactive arthritis and respiratory disorders secondary to aspiration. The stool may contain mucus and (rarely) blood and leukocytes; the latter are present only if there is colonic involvement.

Diagnosis is made by isolation of 4–6 μm oocysts or a positive modified acid-fast stain of the stool. Multiple stool specimens may have to be evaluated to make a diagnosis. In patients with acquired immunodeficiency syndrome (AIDS), oocysts can be isolated from the entire gastrointestinal tract as well as the respiratory and biliary tracts at biopsy or autopsy. Leukocytosis is not common, but eosinophilia has been reported. Radiologic examination of the abdomen is nonspecific, with findings of mucosal folds, air fluid levels, and distended loops of bowel. In patients with biliary tract symptoms, a sonogram should be obtained. The sonogram may show an enlarged gallbladder with thickened walls, dilated intra- and extrahepatic bile ducts, and a normal or stenotic distal common bile duct. Cholangiograms show beading of the common bile duct or papillary stenosis.

Gallbladder carriage of *Cryptosporidium* is chronic, and patients may have to undergo papillotomy, sphincterotomy, cholecystectomy, or T-tube drainage. The prognosis for these patients usually is poor. Histologic examination of the bile and gallbladder shows oocysts along with other organisms such as cytomegalovirus, *Enterobacter cloacae,* and microsporidia.

Therapy includes hospitalization for dehydration, total parenteral nutrition, and correction of electrolyte imbalances. The diarrhea can be relieved with antidiarrheal agents. There is no effective treatment for cryptosporidiosis. Octreotide and paromomycin provide symptomatic improvement of the diarrhea, but do not eradicate the oocysts from the gastrointestinal tract. The oocysts of cryptosporidia are resistant to common disinfectants; therefore, enteric precautions and good handwashing techniques should be used to prevent spread. Patients with human immunodeficiency virus infection and CD$_4$ counts $< 200/\mu$l should only drink boiled or bottled water and avoid infected persons and animals.

The prognosis for AIDS patients with chronic cryptosporidial infection is poor, as recovery depends on the immune status of the host.

In the present patient, cryptosporidia were demonstrated in stained stool specimens. His diarrhea was unresponsive to a variety of anti-infective drugs, and he died 3 months later.

Clinical Pearls

1. Gallbladder infection may occur in 10% of AIDS patients with cryptosporidiosis.

2. Ingestion of only a small number of *Cryptosporidium parvum* oocysts is required to cause infection.

3. There is no effective therapy for cryptosporidiosis, but HIV antivirals have activity against cryptosporidia.

REFERENCES

1. Rubinoff MJ, Field M: Infectious diarrhea. Annu Rev Med 1991; 42:403–410.
2. Wittner M, Tanowitz HB, Weiss LM: Parasitic infections in AIDS patients. Infect Dis Clin North Am 1993; 7:569–586.
3. Centers for Disease Control and Prevention: *Cryptosporidium* infections associated with swimming pools. Dane County, Wisconsin, 1993. MMWR 1994; 43:561–3.
4. Clayton F, Heller T, Kotler DP: Variation in the enteric distribution of cryptosporidia in acquired immunodeficiency syndrome. Am J Clin Pathol 1994; 102:420–425.
5. Ungar BLP: *Cryptosporidium*. In Mandell GL, Douglas RG, Bennett JE (eds): Principles and Practice of Infectious Diseases. New York, Churchill Livingstone, 1995, pp 2000–2010.

PATIENT 68

A 38-year-old man with abdominal pain, fever, and chills

A 38-year-old man presents with a 3-day history of generalized abdominal pain, nausea, vomiting, diarrhea, and fevers to 38.3° C associated with chills. He has a history of nephropathy (related to human immunodeficiency virus [HIV]), hypertension, and end-stage renal disease. The patient is currently on chronic ambulatory peritoneal dialysis (CAPD).

Physical Examination: Temperature 36.8°; pulse 92; respirations 14; blood pressure 180/80. HEENT: no oral thrush, pharynx clear, no lymphadenopathy. Chest: clear to auscultation. Cardiac: regular rate and rhythm, no murmur. Abdomen: soft, diffusely tender, no rebound or guarding, mildly decreased bowel sounds. Extremities: no rashes or edema. Neurologic: no deficits.

Laboratory Findings: Hct 31%; WBC 13,400/μl with 87% granulocytes, 13% lymphocytes. Na^+ 135 mEq/L, K^+ 4.5 mEq/L, Cl^- 84 mEq/L, HCO_3^- 31 mEq/L. BUN 116 mg/dl, creatinine 16.1 mg/dl. Liver function tests: normal. Prothrombin time: 11.1 seconds. Chest radiograph: normal. Semi-quantitative culture of dialysis catheter tip: > 15 cfu/ml gram-negative bacilli (see figure). Peritoneal fluid analysis: 5864/μl leukocytes with moderate quantities of the same gram-negative bacillus.

Question: What is your diagnosis?

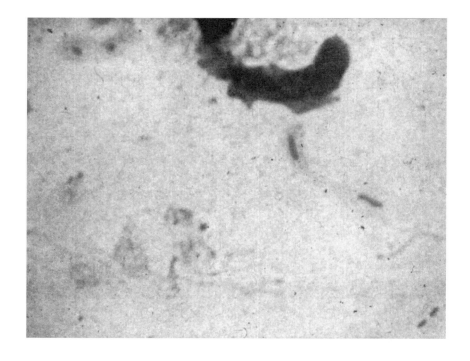

Diagnosis: Peritonitis caused by *Pseudomonas aeruginosa* and intra-abdominal abscess secondary to CAPD catheter

Discussion: Peritonitis associated with chronic ambulatory dialysis most often is caused by endogenous skin flora, catheter exit site and subcutaneous tunnel infections, or contaminated dialysis fluid. *Staphylococcus epidermidis* is the most common cause, followed by *S. aureus,* streptococci, and the diphtheroids. The isolation of enteric gram-negative bacilli suggests fecal contamination or a primary intra-abdominal source. Peritonitis can result from hematogenous spread of alpha hemolytic streptococci, *Mycobacterium tuberculosis,* or ascending infection with pathogens such as *Candida* species from the female genital tract.

Symptoms of peritonitis include abdominal pain, nausea, vomiting, fever, and occasionally diarrhea, which can develop as early as 24 hours after dialysis. Physical examination reveals generalized abdominal tenderness with or without rebound and rigidity. Patients with *S. aureus* peritonitis complain of severe abdominal pain and develop major systemic complications including hypotension, septic shock, and toxic shock syndrome. The presence of palpable, fluctuant abdominal masses may be indicative of large intra-abdominal abscesses.

The diagnosis of bacterial peritonitis is made by a cloudy dialysate with $>100/\mu l$ polymorphonuclear cells and neutrophil predominance ($> 50\%$) on Gram stain and culture in a symptomatic patient. Other laboratory findings include leukocytosis, hemoconcentration, subdiaphragmatic air, and distended loops of bowel. Most patients improve in 1–4 days after initiation of intraperitoneal and/or systemic antibodies. Therapy should be continued for 10 days to 3 weeks depending on clinical improvement and decreased dialysate cell counts.

Persistent symptoms suggest a resistant or unusual organism, inadequate therapy, intra-abdominal perforation, or abscess formation. Computed tomography scan of the abdomen is helpful in identifying abscesses that require percutaneous or surgical drainage.

Peritonitis caused by *P. aeruginosa* is more resistant to treatment and is often associated with multiple abscesses. The catheter should be removed, and combination therapy with two antipseudomonal drugs should be started. In *M. tuberculosis* peritonitis, the dialysate has a lymphocytic pleocytosis, with negative Gram stain and culture results. Diagnosis of *M. tuberculosis* peritonitis requires peritoneal biopsy. HIV-infected patients undergoing CAPD have a high incidence of pseudomonal and candidal peritonitis and experience a high morbidity. They require hospitalization for prolonged antibiotic treatment.

CAPD catheters should be removed within 2 weeks of therapy in patients with CAPD-associated peritonitis complicated by intraperitoneal abscesses, recurrent infection with the same organism, fecal peritonitis, or infections with *P. aeruginosa* fungi or *M. tuberculosis.* The catheters should be replaced only after successful treatment of the peritonitis. CAPD-associated peritonitis can be prevented by adhering to aseptic technique when inserting catheters and during dialysis.

In the present patient, *P. aeruginosa* was repeatedly recovered from the dialysis fluid. Multiple courses of anti-*Pseudomonas* antibiotics failed to clear the infection. Finally, the patient's catheter was removed and replaced with another, and he has since remained free of infection.

Clinical Pearls

1. In peritonitis associated with chronic ambulatory peritoneal dialysis, bacteremia is rare and suggests infection at other sites.

2. The low pH and high osmolarity of peritoneal dialysis fluid are risk factors for peritonitis.

3. Aggressive therapy is required for peritonitis due to *S. aureus, P. aeruginosa,* or fungus because of a tendency for relapse.

REFERENCES

1. Cameron JS: Host defenses in continuous ambulatory peritoneal dialysis and the genesis of peritonitis. Pediatr Nephrol 1995; 9:647–662.
2. Bouza P, Garcia Falcon T, Perez Fontan M, et al: Treatment of CAPD-related peritonitis with ciprofloxacin: Results after 7 years. Adv Perit Dial 1996; 12:185–188.
3. Tzamaloukas AH: Peritonitis in peritoneal dialysis patients: An overview. Adv Ren Replace Ther 1996; 3:232–236.
4. Lai MN, Kao MT, Chen CC, et al: Intraperitoneal once-daily doses of cefazolin and gentamicin for treating CAPD peritonitis. Perit Dial Int 1997; 17:87–89.

PATIENT 69

A 70-year-old patient with fever, cough, pleuritic chest pain, and chills

A 70-year-old man presents to the emergency department complaining of right-sided pleuritic chest pain, cough productive of thick greenish-yellow sputum, increasing dyspnea, fevers, and shaking chills—all of 2-day duration. He denies nausea, vomiting, and diarrhea. His past medical history is significant for chronic obstructive pulmonary disease (COPD), tracheostomy for laryngeal cancer, and alcohol abuse.

Physical Examination: Temperature 38.6°; respirations 26; heart rate 110; blood pressure 140/84. General: ill appearing, but alert and oriented to person, place, and time. HEENT: thick, greenish-yellow sputum from tracheostomy tube. Chest: bilateral scattered rhonchi and bronchial breath sounds, with dullness to percussion and egophony at the right base.

Laboratory Findings: Hct 37%; WBC 15,800/μl with 88% polymorphonuclear cells, 8% bands, 4% lymphocytes. Na$^+$ 138 mEq/L. BUN 32 mg/dl, creatinine 1.2 mg/dl. Arterial blood gas (room air): pH 7.38, PCO$_2$ 22 mmHg, PO$_2$ 78 mmHg. Chest radiograph: right lower lobe opacity with an air bronchogram (see figure). Sputum Gram stain: abundant leukocytes and gram-positive diplococci. Blood cultures: pending.

Question: What is your diagnosis?

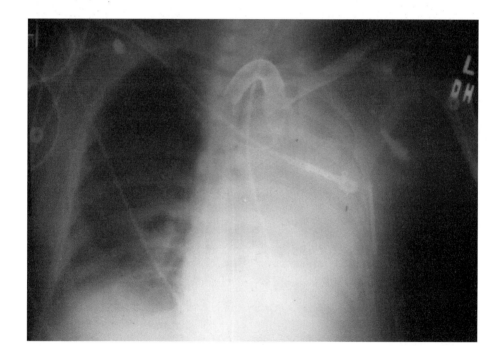

Diagnosis: Pneumococcal pneumonia

Discussion: *Streptococcus pneumoniae* is the most common cause of community-acquired pneumonia. Different serotypes of *S. pneumoniae* normally colonize the upper respiratory tract. In the presence of a viral respiratory infection or after microaspiration of oropharyngeal secretions, these commensals adhere to alveolar cells and cause infection. Risk factors for the development of pneumococcal pneumonia include extremes of age, cigarette smoking, COPD, chronic bronchitis, lung malignancies, asplenism (anatomic or functional), acquired immunodeficiency syndrome, alcoholism, diabetes mellitus, congestive heart failure, and dementia and other neurologic disorders that increase the chances of aspiration.

The presentation of pneumococcal pneumonia varies considerably and is dependent on the age of the patient and underlying risk factors. Most cases develop following an upper respiratory tract (URI) infection. Patients present with worsening URI symptoms and increased sputum production. Classically, the onset of pneumococcal pneumonia is abrupt, with a sudden shaking chill followed by a temperature of 39.4–40.5°C, tachycardia, and tachypnea. Subsequently, patients develop pleuritic chest pain and cough productive of blood-tinged or rusty-colored sputum. Elderly patients may present with mental status changes and hypothermia, but without symptoms of fever, cough, and sputum production. Patients who are chronic smokers and those with COPD notice a sputum color change from white to yellow/green and an increase in production, as well as symptoms of fever, malaise, and worsening dyspnea.

Patients with pneumococcal pneumonia appear acutely ill, with fever, dyspnea, severe pleuritic chest pain, splinting, and tachycardia. Since pneumococcal pneumonia is lobar, bronchial breath sounds are heard on auscultation of the involved lung, with dullness to percussion and increased tactile fremitus and egophony. There also may be abdominal distention secondary to paralytic ileus and acute gastric dilatation. Leukocytosis is present in the majority of cases, but leukopenia is seen in the elderly and in patients with overwhelming infection and bacteremia. Typically, chest radiographs show single or multiple lobar involvement and branching air bronchograms; in the elderly and in immunocompromised patients, opacities may be patchy. Gram stain of the sputum reveals abundant leukocytes with gram-positive diplococci. A positive sputum culture is obtained in only 25–50% of sputum samples.

Twenty to thirty percent of patients with pneumococcal pneumonia have bacteremia, which is a risk factor for a poor clinical outcome. Infectious complications of bacteremia include meningitis, endocarditis, pericarditis, septic arthritis, and peritonitis in patients with ascites. Empyema develops in 1–2% of patients with pneumococcal pneumonia. Pneumococcal lung abscess is rare. Overwhelming infection with disseminated intravascular coagulation and adult respiratory distress syndrome may occur in immunocompromised patients, the elderly, and patients without spleens. Patients with serotype III infection have the worst prognosis. Fatality rates are 25% for untreated pneumococcal pneumonia and 5% for treated cases. The mortality rate of untreated or treated bacteremic pneumococcal pneumonia is four times that of nonbacteremic infection.

Patients clinically improve within 12–36 hours of institution of appropriate therapy, but in some cases 7 days are required. Recovery usually is accompanied by an abrupt defervescence and diaphoresis. Resolution on chest radiograph occurs 8–16 weeks after acute infection subsides. The antibiotic of choice for pneumococcal pneumonia is intravenous penicillin G in daily doses of 1.2–2-4 million units for susceptible isolates with minimal inhibitory concentration (MIC) < 0.1–1.0 μg/ml, or a cephalosporin (ceftriaxone or cefotaxime) for those isolates with MIC > 2.0 μg/ml. Patients should be treated with intravenous antibiotics until afebrile for 3–4 days, then switched to oral therapy to complete a 5- to 10-day course.

Pneumococcal pneumonia can be prevented by administration of the 23-valent polysaccharide vaccine, which includes the serotypes that cause 85–90% of bacteremic infections. It is recommended that the following individuals receive the vaccine: healthy persons age 65 and over; immunocompromised persons with malignancies or human immunodeficiency virus infection; persons with chronic cardiac and pulmonary conditions, asplenia (functional or anatomic), diabetes mellitus, chronic renal insufficiency, cerebrospinal fluid leaks, or alcoholism; and persons in crowded living conditions.

The present patient's sputum and blood cultures were positive for *S. pneumoniae*. He responded to a 14-day course of ceftriaxone.

Clinical Pearls

1. Pleural effusions are uncommon, but empyema is the most common complication of pneumococcal pneumonia.
2. Chest radiograph resolution may take 8–16 weeks.
3. Bacteremia is common in patients with pneumococcal pneumonia.

REFERENCES

1. Farrington M, Rubenstein D: Antigen detection in pneumococcal pneumonia. J Infect 1991; 23:109–116.
2. Friedland IF, McCracken GH Jr: Management of infections caused by antibiotic resistant *Streptococcus pneumoniae*. N Engl J Med 1994; 331:377–382.
3. Guerra LG, Ho H, Verghese A: New pathogens in pneumonia. Med Clin North Am 1994; 78:967–985.
4. Cunha BA: The antibiotic treatment of community-acquired, atypical, and nosocomial pneumonias. Med Clin North Am 1995; 79:581–598.

PATIENT 70

A 45-year-old woman with fever and headache

A 45-year-old woman presents in July with a 2-day history of severe headache associated with photophobia, sore throat, nausea, and diarrhea. She denies fever, chills, vomiting, and rash. There was no improvement in her symptoms on analgesics. The patient's past medical history is unremarkable, and she has no known drug allergies.

Physical Examination: Temperature 38°; pulse 9; respirations 18, blood pressure 100/60. General: mild distress. HEENT: pupils equally round, reactive to light and accommodation; fundi normal, mild conjunctival injection; mild nuchal rigidity of neck; mild erythema of posterior pharynx; Kernig and Brudzinski signs negative; no palpable lymphadenopathy. Abdomen: soft, nontender, normal bowel sounds. Extremities: no rashes or lesions. Neurologic: alert and oriented to person, place, and time; no focal deficits.

Laboratory Findings: WBC 9500/μl with normal differential. Glucose: 88 mg/dl. Cerebrospinal fluid (CSF): clear; glucose 54 mg/dl; RBC 8/μl; WBC 566/μl with 88% lymphocytes, 1% neutrophils, 11% monocytes. Gram stain: numerous WBCs but no organisms (see figure). Urinalysis: normal.

Questions: What is the most likely diagnosis? What additional tests would you order?

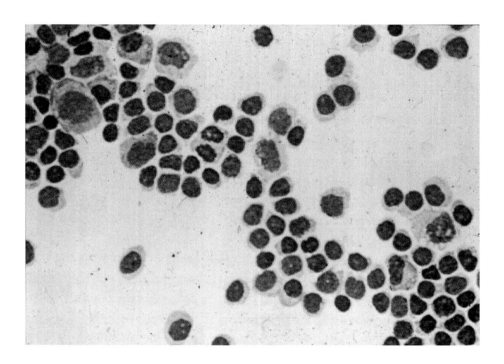

Diagnosis: Enteroviral aseptic meningitis

Discussion: Aseptic (viral) meningitis is a clinical syndrome with short-term morbidity caused by the non-polio enteroviruses, which include groups A and B coxsackieviruses, echoviruses, and enteroviruses 68–71. These enteroviruses are able to cause a spectrum of central nervous system (CNS) infections ranging from mild to severe aseptic meningitis to encephalitis and myelitis. The spectrum and severity of clinical disease varies with age, gender, immune status of the affected individual, and the virulence of the enteroviral serotype. The enteroviruses most commonly isolated from clinical specimens of patients with aseptic meningitis are coxsackie B serotypes 1–5 and echovirus serotypes 4, 6, 9, 11, 16, and 30. Non-polio enteroviruses account for 80–90% of all cases of aseptic meningitis for which an etiologic agent is identified. Children and adults less than 40 years old are most commonly affected.

Infection is acquired by the fecal oral route or via respiratory droplet secretions. After the virus enters the gastrointestinal tract, it replicates and causes initially a mild and then a significant viremia, with signs and symptoms of viral infection. Many organ systems are seeded during viremia, including the CNS, liver, lungs, and heart. The ability to clear the enterovirus is antibody-mediated, and patients who are agammaglobulinemic and neonates (who usually acquire infection perinatally) have severe illness with increased morbidity and mortality. Aseptic meningitis has a benign clinical course, and should be recognized as a syndrome of meningeal irritation and CSF pleocytosis when there is no evidence of encephalitis or myelitis.

More than 75,000 cases of enteroviral aseptic meningitis are reported in the United States every year, particularly in the summer and fall months, with peak incidence in late summer and early fall. Seasonal outbreaks may occur. The onset may be gradual or abrupt and is usually biphasic. Patients present initially with nonspecific signs and symptoms of a viral infection—fever, vomiting, anorexia, fine maculopapular rash, cough, pharyngitis, diarrhea, and myalgia—which resolve. Two to ten days later, headache, fever at 38–40°C, nuchal rigidity, and photophobia acutely develop. Nuchal rigidity presents in only 50% of patients and varies from mild to severe. Kernig and Brudzinzki signs are present in only 30% of adults.

Focal neurologic findings are rare, occurring in 5–10% of patients early in the course of the disease. They include febrile seizures in children, complex seizures, lethargy, coma, and movement disorders.

Focal neurologic symptoms resolve slowly, and their presence suggests encephalitis or myelitis due to enteroviruses and other neurotropic viruses, e.g., herpes simplex, arbovirus, and mumps viruses. In patients presenting with evidence of encephalitis, petechial rash, and muscle weakness, other diagnoses to be considered include polio virus, partially treated bacterial or meningococcal meningitis, acute human immunodeficiency virus infection, and Lyme borreliosis. In patients with asceptic meningitis, fever and signs of meningeal irritation subside in approximately 3–7 days. Agammaglobulinemic patients may have chronic aseptic meningitis or meningoencephalitis lasting for many years. Patients should undergo lumbar puncture to exclude bacterial meningitis. The CSF in aseptic meningitis is clear under normal or slightly increased pressure. The cell count is 10–500/μl with polymorphonuclear predominance and mononuclear shift after 1–2 days, and the count may persist for 1 week or more after fever and signs of meningeal irritation have resolved. The glucose is normal; the protein is normal or slightly elevated; and the Gram stain is negative. The peripheral white blood cell count can be low, normal, or elevated, with a normal differential or left shift.

The ability to culture enteroviruses from the CSF, nasopharynx, throat, and feces within the first week of onset of meningitis helps confirm the diagnosis. Isolation of the virus in cell culture is the gold standard for diagnosis, but may take 4–10 days. Detection of the virus by polymerase chain reaction is a much faster method, providing a diagnosis in 48 hours. If the CSF results suggest aseptic meningitis (i.e., CSF pleocytosis and negative Gram stain), patients can be observed and treated symptomatically. There is no need to repeat the lumbar puncture. There is no recommended antiviral therapy. Hospitalization is not necessary, except in sporadic cases or when a diagnosis of bacterial meningitis or viral encephalitis is being considered. Children or adults with compromised humoral immunity should be treated with intravenous, intrathecal, or intraventricular gamma globulin. Neonates with overwhelming sepsis have been treated with intravenous gamma globulin, maternal plasma, and exchange transfusions.

The present patient exhibited mild meningitic symptoms. Her CSF showed no evidence of bacterial meningitis. Coxsackievirus grew from viral cultures of her throat and stool. Her symptoms slowly resolved after 10 days with symptomatic treatment.

Clinical Pearls

1. The clinical course of aseptic meningitis in adults is benign and short-lived.

2. Nonsteroidal anti-inflammatory drugs, particularly ibuprofen, are not an uncommon cause of aseptic meningitis.

3. Neonates are at highest risk for severe clinical illness complicated by meningoencephalitis.

4. The CSF lactic acid levels are the best rapid test to differentiate viral/aseptic meningitis from partially treated/bacterial meningitis.

5. All patients suspected of having meningitis should have a lumbar puncture for diagnosis.

REFERENCES

1. Hammer SM, Connolly KJ: Viral aseptic meningitis in the United States: Clinical features, viral etiologies, and differential diagnosis. Curr Clin Topics Infect Dis 1992; 12:1–25.
2. Modlin JF: Coxsackieviruses, echoviruses, and newer enteroviruses. In Mandell GL, Douglas RG, Bennett JE (eds): Principles and Practice of Infectious Diseases. New York, Churchill Livingstone, 1995, pp 1620–1636.
3. Rotbart HA: Enteroviral infections of the central nervous system. Clin Infect Dis 1995; 20:971–981.
4. Cunha BA: The diagnostic significance of the CSF lactic acid. Infect Dis Practice 1997; 21:57–60.
5. Zuckerman D, Chua A, Cunha BA: Enteroviral meningitis. Emergency Med 1997; 29:109–113.

PATIENT 71

A 12-year-old girl with fever, strawberry tongue, truncal rash, and peripheral edema

A 12-year-old girl is brought to the emergency department with a 3-day history of fevers to 39.4°C, abdominal pain, diarrhea, and anorexia. She also has a rash that started on the trunk, palms, and soles and is associated with swelling of the hands and feet. She denies headache, neck stiffness, and photophobia. There is no history of recent travel or insect bites. The family has a pet dog.

Physical Examination: Temperature 38.3°; pulse 140; respirations 20; blood pressure 80/60. General: lethargic. Skin: erythematous maculopapular rash on face, trunk, and extremities, including palms and soles (see figure). HEENT: bilateral injection of the conjunctivae, mild periobital edema, strawberry tongue, supple neck with mild anterior lymphadenopathy. Chest: clear to auscultation. Cardiac: normal, no murmur. Abdomen: soft, nontender, normal bowel sounds. Extremities: bilateral edema of hands and feet. Neurologic: no deficits.

Laboratory Findings: Hct 36%; WBC 16,800/μl with 86% polymorphonuclear cells, 2% bands, 12% lymphocytes; platelets 234,000/μl; hemoglobin 12 mg/dl. Chest radiograph: normal. Urinalysis: normal.

Questions: What is the suspected diagnosis? How would you manage this patient?

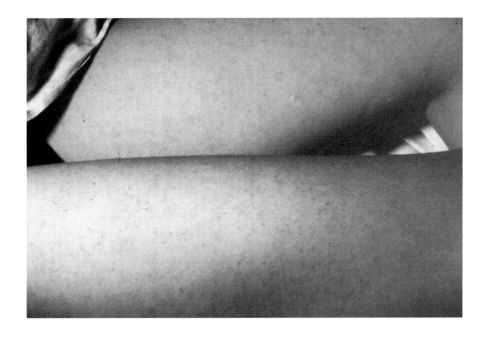

Diagnosis: Kawasaki disease

Discussion: Kawasaki disease is an acute, multisystemic vasculitis of unknown etiology involving small- and medium-sized arteries. The disease affects children ages 2 months to 5 years and is rare after age 12. Males are affected more often than females. The disease does not appear to have an infectious etiology. Peak incidence is in the winter and spring. Kawasaki disease is found worldwide, and is the most common cause of acquired heart disease in children in the United States.

The diagnostic criteria for Kawasaki disease includes fever of at least 5-day duration plus four additional symptoms: rash, bilateral conjunctivitis, changes of the lips and oral mucosa, changes of the extremities, or cervical adenopathy. The acute febrile illness can last 1–2 weeks. Patients present with fevers > 39°C, irritability, lethargy, colicky abdominal pain, diarrhea, and anorexia. Within 24 hours, an erythematous polymorphous rash appears on the trunk and perineum. The rash is followed a few days later by bilateral conjunctival injection (nonpurulent conjunctivitis); mucous membrane changes with dry, red-fissured lips; red strawberry tongue; and an injected pharynx. Erythema or a purplish-red discoloration and edema of the palms and soles appear on days 3–5. Cervical lymphadenopathy is not prominent.

Two to four weeks after the onset of acute febrile illness, the fever, rash, and lymphadenopathy resolve and periungual, palmar, and plantar desquamation occurs. However, cardiac complications manifest during this period, coinciding with a significant thrombocytosis which can be >1,000,000/μl platelets. The cardiac complications include coronary artery aneurysms (occurring in 20% of patients), pericarditis, myocarditis, myocardial ischemia, myocardial infarction, dysrhythmias, cardiomegaly, mitral or aortic insufficiency, and sudden death. *Cardiac involvement is the hallmark of Kawasaki disease.* All patients with Kawasaki disease should have a baseline echocardiogram, repeated 3–6 weeks later.

Beau's lines (transverse grooves) appear across the fingernails 8–12 weeks after the onset of symptoms. Leukocytosis, thrombocytosis, and the erythrocyte sedimentation rate (elevated during the acute febrile illness) return to normal values 6–10 weeks into convalescence.

Noncardiac features of Kawasaki disease include arthralgia, arthritis, sterile pyuria, urethritis, aseptic meningitis, obstructive jaundice, hydrops of the gallbladder, pneumonitis, peripheral ischemia, gangrene, and sensorineural hearing loss.

Kawasaki disease is unresponsive to antibiotic therapy. Therapy includes high-dose, intravenous immunoglobulin (IVIG) within the first 10 days to decrease fever, symptoms of acute febrile illness, and risk of developing coronary artery aneurysms. IVIG is given as a single infusion dose of 2g/kg over 10 hours. Aspirin also should be given during the first 2 weeks of illness. In patients without coronary artery disease, aspirin should be continued until the platelet count returns to normal. In patients with coronary artery aneurysms, aspirin should be continued indefinitely, or until aneurysms resolve. Recurrence of Kawasaki disease is rare, presenting in 3–5% of patients about 3 months after the initial illness.

The present patient had an uncomplicated course of Kawasaki disease and responded well to IVIG and aspirin therapy.

Clinical Pearls

1. Cardiac involvement is the hallmark of Kawasaki disease.

2. The rash of Kawasaki disease predominantly involves the trunk and perineum, but the face and extremities also can be affected.

3. Inflammatory arthritis involving the large joints, i.e., knees and ankles, usually occurs 10 days after the onset of illness.

REFERENCES

1. Rauch A, Hurwitz E: Centers for Disease Control case definition of Kawasaki syndrome. Pediatr Infect Dis J 1985; 4:702–703.
2. Rose V: Kawasaki syndrome: Cardiovascular manifestations. J Rheumatol 1990; 17(Suppl 24):11–14.
3. Rowley AH, Shulman ST: Current therapy for acute Kawasaki syndrome. J Pediatr 1991; 118:987–991.
4. Kawasaki T: Kawasaki disease. Acta Pediatr 1995; 84:713–715.

PATIENT 72

A 39-year-old man with acquired immunodeficiency syndrome, dypsnea, nonproductive cough, and bilateral interstitial opacities

A 39-year-old man presents to the emergency department with a 4-day history of worsening dyspnea, fevers to 38.3°C, shaking chills, and a nonproductive cough that has been worsening over the previous 2 weeks. He also complains of anorexia and a 5-pound weight loss in the last week. He denies abdominal pain, diarrhea, and recent travel. The patient is HIV positive, and his last CD_4 count (2 years ago) was 350/μl. He has no known drug allergies.

Physical Examination: Temperature 38.6°; pulse 114; respirations 42; blood pressure 142/82. General: moderate respiratory distress. HEENT: thrush on buccal mucosa; otherwise normal. Chest: bilateral coarse breath sounds.

Laboratory Findings: Arterial blood gas (room air): pH 7.44, PCO_2 23 mmHg, PO_2 52 mmHg, SaO_2 78%. Chest radiograph: bilateral interstitial and alveolar opacities. Bronchoscopy with bronchoalveolar lavage: results pending.

Questions: What is your diagnosis? How would you pursue it?

Diagnosis: Pneumonia caused by *Pneumocystis carinii*

Discussion: *Pneumocystis carinii* is the most common cause of pneumonia in patients infected with human immunodeficiency virus (HIV) who have T-helper cell or CD_4 counts of $< 200/\mu l$. The lower the count, the higher the risk for acquiring infection. Immunocompromised patients acquire *Pneumocystis carinii* by inhalation of airborne aerosols from persons with active disease. The organism incubates in the alveoli for 4–8 weeks before causing symptoms, which can last from weeks to months. Patients present with fever, progressive dyspnea, and nonproductive cough. Other symptoms include weight loss, fatigue, chest pain, and chills.

Tachypnea and fever are the most common findings on physical examination. In 50% of patients, auscultation of the lungs is normal; in the remainder, rales or rhonchi may be present. Room air blood gas shows hypoxemia, $O_2 < 70$ mmHg, respiratory alkalosis, and an alveolar-oxygen [P(A-a)O_2] gradient widened with the severity of disease. LDH is elevated in 90% of patients with *P. carinii* pneumonia (PCP). Pulmonary function tests show a restrictive-type pattern, with decreased vital capacity and total lung capacity.

Severity of Disease	P(A-a) O_2
Mild	< 35
Moderate	35–45
Severe	> 45

Diagnosis is made by finding cysts in sputum or bronchoalveolar lavage specimens that stain with Gram Weigert or Grocott-Gomori (methenamine silver nitrate). Chest radiographs are normal in 5–10% of symptomatic patients. The typical chest radiograph findings are bilateral, interstitial, or alveolar opacities. Other radiographic findings include unilateral opacities, nodules, cavities, pneumatoceles, and lymphadenopathy. Pleural effusions are rare. Apical opacities, cysts, and pneumathoraces are seen in patients who develop PCP while on aerosolized pentamidine prophylaxis.

Extrapulmonary PCP involving other organ systems is seen in patients with endstage AIDS who have not received PCP prophylaxis or are on aerosolized pentamidine prophylaxis. Trimethoprim-sulfamethoxazole (TMP-SMX; 15–20 mg/kg/day TMP plus 75–100 mg/kg/day SMX) in four divided doses, and pentamidine isethionate (4 mg/kg/day) in one dose are the drugs of choice for the initial treatment of mild to severe PCP. Adjunctive therapy with corticosteroids in tapering doses is recommended for the treatment of moderate to severe disease to decrease the risk of respiratory failure and death.

Day of Therapy	Prednisone Dose
1–5	40 mg bid
6–10	40 mg qd
11–20	20 mg qd

Eighty to ninety percent of patients treated with TMP-SMX develop side effects while taking the medication. These include fever, rash, neutropenia, thrombocytopenia, and hepatitis. For patients who cannot tolerate either TMP-SMX or pentamidine, other therapies are trimetrexate plus leucovorin for all stages of desease; and atavaquone alone or combination therapy with trimethoprim plus dapsone, primaquine, or clindamycin for mild to moderate disease.

PCP in AIDS should be treated with any of the above therapies for 21 days. Institution of therapy should not be delayed if bronchoalveolar lavage is not immediately available. Primary prophylaxis for PCP is recommended for all patients who are HIV positive with a CD_4 count $< 200/\mu l$ or are rapidly deteriorating clinically. Secondary prophylaxis is recommended for all patients who have recovered from an episode of PCP. Patients should receive 1) oral TMP-SMX DS one tablet every day or three times a week, or 2) oral dapsone, 100 mg once a day, or 3) aerosolized pentamidine, 300 mg every 4 weeks via Respigard jet nebulizer.

The prognosis for AIDS patients with PCP depends on the degree of hypoxemia and the immunocompromised state of the host. Without secondary prophylaxis, 60% of patients relapse within the first year. Symptoms may be milder and the chest radiograph findings atypical. There is no acquired immunity to PCP.

Clinical Pearls

1. Pleural effusions are rare in pneumonia due to *Pneumocystis carinii*.
2. Extrapulmonary PCP is seen in patients with endstage AIDS who are on aerosolized pentamidine prophylaxis or have not received any prophylaxis.

REFERENCES

1. Gagnon S, Boota AM, Fischl MA, et al: Corticosteroids as adjunctive therapy for severe *Pneumocystis carinii* pneumonia in acquired immune deficiency syndrome. N Engl J Med 1990; 323:1444–1450.
2. Phair J, Muñoz A, Detels R, et al: The risk of *Pneumocystis carinii* pneumonia among men infected with the human immunodeficiency virus type 1. Multicenter AIDS Cohort Study Group. N Engl J Med 1990; 322:161–165.
3. Smith D, Gazzard B: Treatment and prophylaxis of *Pneumocystis carinii* pneumonia in AIDS patients. Drug 1991; 42:628–639.
4. Hoover DR, Saah AJ, Bacellar H, et al: Clinical manifestations of AIDS in the era of pneumocystis prophylaxis. N Engl J Med 1993; 329:1922–1926.
5. Moe AA, Hardy WD: *Pneumocystis carinii* infection in the HIV-seropositive patient. Infect Dis Clin North Am 1994; 8:331–364.
6. Rosen MJ: Pneumonia in patients with HIV infection. Med Clin North Am 1994; 78:1067–1079.

PATIENT 73

A 20-year-old homosexual man with bloody diarrhea and abdominal pain

A 20-year-old homosexual man presents with a 3-day history of bloody diarrhea, tenesmus, crampy lower abdominal pain, fever to 39.5°C, and chills. He admits to having multiple sexual partners but has never been tested for human immunodeficiency virus.

Physical Examination: Temperature 39.6°; pulse 126; respirations 24. General: cachectic and lethargic, with dehydrated appearance. HEENT: tongue coated, thrush on buccal mucosa; palpable lymphadenopathy. Chest: clear bilaterally. Abdomen: mildly distended with bilateral lower quadrant tenderness and hyperactive bowel sounds, no hepatosplenomegaly. Rectal: blood-tinged mucus; stool has "currant jelly" appearance (see figure). Skin: no rashes. Chest radiograph: normal. Abdominal radiograph: distended loops of bowel.

Laboratory Examination: WBC 23,000/μl with 62% polymorphonuclear cells, 22% bands, 16% lymphocytes. Na$^+$ 124 mEq/L, Cl$^-$ 109 mEq/L, HCO$_3^-$ 18 mEq/L. BUN 40 mg/dl, creatinine 1.2 mg/dl, glucose 63 mg/dl. Stool Gram stain and blood cultures: pending.

Questions: What is the cause of the patient's present condition? How would you initiate therapy?

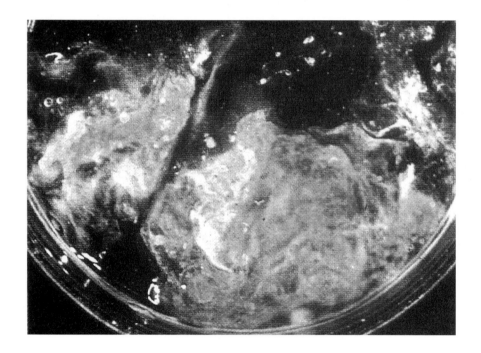

Diagnosis: Shigellosis

Discussion: *Shigella* species are gram-negative, nonmotile, nonencapsulated bacteria that are the most easily transmissible agents of the infectious diarrheas worldwide. The severity of diarrhea and bacillary dysentery is determined by the infecting species. *Shigella dysenteriae* and *Shigella flexneri* have caused worldwide epidemics of bacillary dysentery associated with high mortality rates and, very rarely, shigellemia in malnourished and immunocompromised persons. *Shigella sonnei* and *Shigella boydii* cause a self-limited, watery diarrhea. *S. sonnei* is the most commonly isolated species in cases of shigellosis in the United States and industrialized countries. The most commonly affected group is children aged 6 months to 10 years. *Shigella* species are natural human pathogens, transmitted from person to person by the fecal-oral route, especially in crowded, unsanitary conditions and by ingestion of contaminated food and water. Male homosexuals serve as a major reservoir for these organisms.

Shigellosis is an acute diarrheal illness with symptoms of systemic toxicity. Only a few of these fastidious organisms are required to transmit disease, because they are able to withstand the acidity of the stomach and lodge in the small and then large intestine, where they replicate. Initially, crampy abdominal pain develops, with fevers as high as 41.1°C and massive, watery diarrhea up to 30 times a day. These symptoms are followed by lower quadrant tenderness; small-volume stools consisting of blood, mucus, and pus; fecal urgency; tenesmus; and low-grade fevers.

Prolonged infection in malnourished children and the elderly can lead to severe dehydration and death from diarrhea and vomiting, metabolic derangements with severe hyponatremia (sodium 110–120 mEq/L), inappropriate secretion of antidiuretic hormone, and hypoglycemia. Seizures, obtundation, and coma also can complicate the course. Rectal prolapse, toxic colonic dilatation, intestinal perforation, and death can occur with all *Shigella* species, but are most commonly reported with *S. dysenteriae*. Another complication is bacteremia, which is associated with high mortality and is common in children less than 1 year old and in malnourished, immunocompromised persons. Shigella bacteremia rarely has been reported in persons with acquired immunodeficiency syndrome. The few cases typically featured *S. dysenteriae* and *S. flexneri*. Hemolytic uremic syndrome can complicate the course in patients infected with Shiga toxin, which produces *S. dysenteriae* type 1. Post-*Shigella* Reiter's syndrome is not uncommon.

The best way to culture the stool is at the bedside, by directly inoculating the blood or mucus onto selective media. Direct stool examination reveals numerous sheets of polymorphonuclear leukocytes. However, stool cultures are not always positive. Blood cultures should be obtained in toxic patients. If untreated, bacillary dysentery lasts for about 1 week, but symptoms can persist for a month. Antibiotic therapy shortens the duration of symptoms and decreases the number of organisms excreted during episodes. Patients should receive a 3- to 5-day course of oral TMP-SMX or a fluoroquinolone. Intravenous therapy with fluoroquinolone or a third-generation cephalosporin should be started in severely ill patients and the immunocompromised. In dehydrated patients, intravenous fluid losses should be replaced and metabolic derangements corrected.

The present patient was empirically started on an intravenous fluoroquinolone and metronidazole because of the initial presumptive diagnosis of infectious diarrhea. Stool and blood cultures grew *S. flexneri* 2 days later. His CD_4 count was 14. The patient died 4 days after admission.

Clinical Pearls

1. *Shigella* bacteremia is rare and is usually associated with an immunocompromised state.
2. Stool cultures are usually positive in the acute illness.
3. Empiric therapy for shigellosis is a 3- to 5-day course of oral TMP/SMX, or a fluoroquinolone in adults, to shorten the duration of the illness.

Differential Diagnosis of *Shigella* Dysentery

	Shigella Dysentery	Amebic Dysentery	*Salmonella* Infection
Signs and Symptoms			
Onset	Acute	Insidious/abrupt	Subacute
Incubation period	≤ 24 hours	20–90 days	8–48 hours
Vomiting/nausea	Absent	Absent	Common
Fever	Common	Common	Common
Shaking chills	Multiple chills common	No chills	Single initial chill
Tenesmus	Common/severe	Uncommon/mild	Uncommon/mild
Abdominal pain	Severe and maximal over sigmoid/RLQ	Cecal tenderness	Generalized
Stools			
Gross			
Odor	Odorless	Odor of decomposing blood	Foul (H_2S)
Blood	Large amounts	Small amounts	Little or none
pH	↑	↓	N pH
Color	Red currant jelly or colorless	Brown	Dark green or brown
Microscopic			
PMNs	Many clumped PMNs	Few PMNs	Many PMNs
RBCs	Many discrete RBCs	Clumped RBCs	Few discrete RBCs
Bacteria	Few nonmotile bacilli	Many motile bacilli	Many motile bacilli
Sigmoidoscopy (ulcer appearance)	Serpiginous with rough edges	Oval with smooth overhanging edges (flask-shaped)	None

RLQ = right lower quadrant, PMN − polymorphonuclear cell, RBC = red blood cell
From Cunha BA: *Shigella*. Infect Dis Practice 1985; 8:1–8. With permission.

REFERENCES

1. Baskin DH, Lax JD, Barenberg D: *Shigella* bacteremia in patients with acquired immunodeficiency syndrome. Am J Gastroenterol 1987; 82:338–341.
2. Heubner J, Czerwenka W, Gruner E, von Graevenitz A: Shigellemia in AIDS patients: Case report and review of the literature. Infection 1993; 21:122–124.

PATIENT 74

A 55-year-old man with fever, erythema, and purulent drainage
from the right leg

A 55-year-old man complains of fevers up to 38.3° C, worsening erythema, and purulent drainage from the lower medial aspect of his right leg. Symptoms commenced 4 days previously. His leg was injured at the same site in an automobile accident 5 years ago. He denies history of diabetes mellitus and is not taking any medication.

Physical Examination: Temperature 38°; pulse 86; respirations 16; blood pressure 142/82. General: well-developed, well-nourished man. Extremities: medial aspect of right lower leg swollen, erythematous, warm, and tender, with purulent drainage from a small opening. Chest: normal. Cardiac: unremarkable. HEENT: normal.

Laboratory Findings: WBC 14,800/µl with 83% polymorphonuclear cells, 16% lymphocytes, 1% monocytes; ESR 76 mm/hr. Gram stain of wound drainage: gram-positive cocci in clusters; identification pending. Blood cultures: negative. Computed tomography scan of right leg: see figure.

Question: What is your diagnosis?

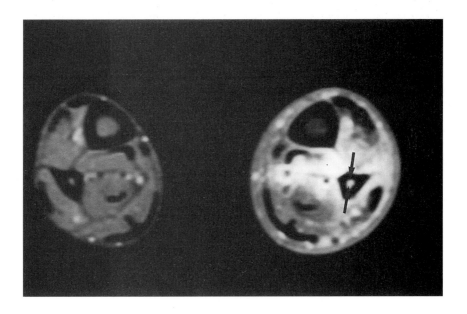

Diagnosis: Osteomyelitis due to *Staphylococcus aureus*

Discussion: Osteomyelitis is classified as acute or chronic depending on the clinical presentation and the radiologic and histologic findings. It also can be defined as hematogenous, secondary to a contiguous focus of infection, or associated with peripheral vascular insufficiency. Anatomically, osteomyelitis can be described as medullary, superficial, localized, or diffuse, depending on the extent of bony involvement. Acute hematogenous osteomyelitis is seen in children, but is uncommon in adults. It usually involves the vertebrae and rarely the long bones of the lower extremities. When the lower extremity is involved, affected areas are the metaphysis in children and the diaphysis in adults.

Immunocompromised persons and intravenous drug abusers are at highest risk for acquiring **acute hematogenous osteomyelitis** with bacteremic spread of infection, which can penetrate the cortical bone and lead to a soft tissue abscess. **Chronic hematogenous osteomyelitis** is more common than acute, and runs a protracted clinical course with recurrent reactivations of a quiescent focus and the eventual formation of sinus tracts. Osteomyelitis in adults typically is a result of a contiguous focus of infection secondary to trauma; nosocomial infection acquired during surgical procedures; insertion of a prosthesis; or spread from an overlying infected wound. By the time it presents, it usually is chronic. In an acute exacerbation of chronic osteomyelitis, patients present with fever, increased pain, swelling, and purulent drainage from an ulceration or sinus tract.

Patients may or may not have leukocytosis, but the erythrocyte sedimentation rate usually is elevated, and this finding can be used to monitor therapy. The purulent drainage should be cultured, and blood cultures should be drawn on all patients suspected of hematogenous osteomyelitis. The differential diagnosis of osteomyelitis includes malignant and benign tumors, past trauma, and bone infarcts from hemaglobulinopathies. Radiographs should be obtained in all patients suspected of osteomyelitis. If the initial images are normal they should be repeated within 2 weeks, because the radiographic changes of osteomyelitis generally are delayed.

Typical findings in acute osteomyelitis include soft tissue swelling, periosteal thickening or elevation, and lytic changes. In chronic osteomyelitis, typical findings are sclerotic bone and periosteal reaction. Indium-labeled scans are useful for delineating the extent of bony destruction in acute osteomyelitis. However, magnetic resonance imaging (MRI) is the most sensitive test for chronic osteomyelitis. The pathogen most frequently isolated in hematogenous osteomyelitis is *Staphylococcus aureus*. Other organisms associated with the disorder include *S. epidermidis, Streptococcus pyogenes, Enterococcus* species, gram-negative bacilli, and anaerobes.

For chronic osteomyelitis, antibiotic treatment can be based on the results of bone, soft tissue, or blood cultures. Cultures should be obtained before antibiotic therapy is started or after the patient has been off antibiotics for 24–48 hours. In the treatment of chronic osteomyelitis, both antibiotics and surgical debridement are necessary for cure. At debridement, all necrotic bone and soft tissue should be removed, and antibiotic therapy should be based on the susceptibility of the organism isolated from bone cultures or deep bone biopsy. The patient should receive parenteral antibiotic therapy to complete a 4-week course after the last curative surgical debridement. Superficial osteomyelitis can be treated with a 2–4 week course of antibiotics after superficial debridement and flap surgery.

The present patient was admitted to the hospital and started on antibiotics for an acute exacerbation of cellulitis over chronically infected bone. Radiographs and MRI showed chronic osteomyelitis of the right tibia. Two weeks later, he underwent debridement of the involved bone, cultures of which grew *S. aureus*. The patient received a 6-week course of antibiotics.

Clinical Pearls

1. Acute hematogeneous osteomyelitis affecting the long bones is rare in adults.

2. In acute osteomyelitis, radiographic changes may be delayed and may actually show worsening although the patient is clinically improving.

3. The most common symptom of osteomyelitis is pain in the area of infection.

4. Acute osteomyelitis may be cured by antibiotics alone. Chronic osteomyelitis requires surgical debridement of infected bone for cure, and antibiotics are ancillary.

REFERENCES

1. Waldvogel FA, Medoff G, Swartz MN: Osteomyelitis: A review of clinical features, therapeutic considerations, and unusual aspects. N Engl J Med 1970; 282:198–206, 260–266, 316–322.
2. Waldvogel FA, Vasey H: Osteomyelitis: The past decade. N Engl J Med 1980; 303:360–370.
3. Mader JT, Calhoun J: Long bone osteomyelitis: Diagnosis and management. Hosp Practice 1994; 29:71–86.

PATIENT 75

A 30-year-old woman with fever, "sunburn" rash, diarrhea, and hypotension

A 30-year-old woman was in her usual state of health until 5 days prior to admission when she experienced mild chills, followed 3 days later by nonspecific vaginal irritation, fever, and sore throat. One day prior to admission, she awoke from sleep with shaking chills and fever of 40°C, nausea, vomiting, and diarrhea. She decided to come to the emergency department after noticing a generalized rash and experiencing a syncopal episode, photophobia, and neck stiffness. Her last menstrual period was 2 weeks ago.

Physical Examination: Temperature 38.5; pulse 136; respirations 28; blood pressure 110/60. General: alert and oriented to person, place, and time; in moderate distress. Cardiac: normal. Skin: warm with a diffuse, erythematous rash over the face, trunk, and extremities (see figure showing right inner arm). Vagina: hyperemic with scattered vesicular lesions.

Laboratory Findings: WBC 12,300/μl with 72% polymorphonuclear cells, 20% bands, 3% lymphocytes, 5% monocytes. BUN 31 mg/dl, creatinine 3.2 mg/dl. Arterial blood gas (room air): pH 7.4, CO_2 30 mmHg, O_2 78 mmHg, SaO_2 96%, HCO_3^- 18 mEq/L. Chest radiograph: bilateral diffuse opacities.

Question: What is your diagnosis?

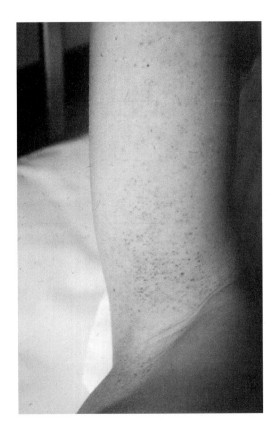

Diagnosis: Toxic shock syndrome

Discussion: Toxic shock syndrome (TSS) is a multisystem disease induced by the pyogenic exotoxins of *Staphylococcus aureus,* TSS toxin 1 (TSST-1), and the enterotoxins A-G. TSST-1 is associated with 65% of TSS—90% of menstrual and 40% of nonmenstrual cases. Enterotoxin B is associated with 20% of cases—0% of menstrual and 40% of nonmenstrual cases. The majority (85%) of TSS cases are associated with the use of highly absorbent tampons by menstruating women. Fifteen percent of TSS cases occur in nonmenstruating women, children, and men. These cases have been associated with the contraceptive sponge, surgical procedures, abortions, childbirth, nonpostpartum vaginal infections, and cutaneous and subcutaneous infections.

In postoperative TSS, patients become symptomatic 2–4 days after surgery without any clinical evidence of wound infection or local inflammation. The onset of postpartum TSS can be early or late, occurring 3–14 days after delivery. Nonpostpartum TSS is associated with vaginal infections and contraceptive use. Menstrual TSS occurs at the onset or within 2 days of the menstrual period.

TSS also is caused by *Streptococcus pyogenes,* which produces streptococcal pyogenic exotoxins (SPEs). Rarely, streptococcal TSS can develop as a complication of pharyngitis, minor nonpenetrating trauma, and surgical procedures, and after varicella and influenza infections. Patients present with severe, painful soft tissue infection, and multiorgan dysfunction develops within 24–72 hours. Coagulase-negative staphylococci, which produce TSST-1, also can cause TSS. Patients with *S. aureus* TSS complain of a prodrome with sudden onset of fever > 38.8° C, nausea, and vomiting and/or watery diarrhea. Severe myalgia may develop within 12–48 hours of the acute illness. This phase is characterized by severe hypotension with hypovolemic shock and syncope; a diffuse, erythematous, macular or petechial or "sunburn" rash, which almost always is present within the first 24 hours; diffuse hyperemia of the mucous membranes; disorientation without focal neurologic findings; oliguria; and hypoxemia. The severity of TSS varies from a mild illness to a life-threatening one requiring intensive care monitoring.

The presence of six of the above criteria in a patient suspected to have TSS makes the diagnosis definite. The diagnosis is probable if only five are present. Other potentially fatal clinical syndromes that resemble TSS—such as streptococcal infection, rickettsiosis, Rocky Mountain spotted fever, leptospirosis, Kawasaki disease, meningococcemia, and rubeola—must be ruled out.

In all cases of menstrual TSS, the vaginal dis-

Criteria for the Diagnosis of TSS

Temperature	> 38.9°C (102°F)
Systolic blood pressure	< 90 mmHg
Erythematous rash that desquamates on the palms and soles during convalescence (1–2 weeks after cessation of illness)	
Involvement of three or more organ systems:	
Gastrointestinal	Vomiting and profuse diarrhea
Muscular	Severe myalgia or increase (> 2× normal) in serum creatinine
Mucous membranes	Vaginal, oropharyngeal, and conjunctival hyperemia
Renal	2× increase in BUN and creatinine over normal upper limit and/or sterile pyuria
Liver	Total bilirubin, aspartate aminotransferase, alanine aminotransferase at least 2× normal upper limit
Hematologic	Thrombocytopenia, < 100,000 platelets/μl
Central nervous system	Alterations in consciousness without focal neurologic findings, evidence of meningeal irritation with sterile cerebrospinal fluid
Cardiopulmonary	Hypoxemia, adult respiratory distress syndrome or depressed myocardial function
Metabolic	Hypocalcemia (serum calcium < 7.0 mg/dl), hypophosphatemia (serum phosphate < 2.5 mg/dl), hypoalbuminemia (serum protein < 5.0 mg/dl)

charge should be cultured. In nonmenstrual TSS, *S. aureus* can be cultured from apparently uninfected wounds. Blood cultures are invariably positive for *S. aureus*. Treatment of TSS includes rapid and aggressive fluid resuscitation, removal of the tampon if present, correction of electrolyte imbalances, exploration and debridement of any surgical wounds or underlying abscesses, and monitoring in an intensive care setting. The patient should be treated with an antistaphylococcal antibiotic for at least 2 weeks.

Although 90% of the general population has antibodies of TSST-1, they are not detectable in early menstruation-associated TSS. Complications of TSS include memory loss, difficulty concentrating, and recurrence within 3 months of the initial menstrual-associated episode. The mortality rate of TSS is 5–10%.

The present patient has nonmenstrual, nonpostpartum TSS associated with a vaginal infection. Vaginal and cervical cultures grew *S. aureus* positive for TSST-1 and negative for enterotoxin B. She had no antibodies to TSST-1 and blood cultures were negative. Two weeks of antistaphylococcal antibiotics restored the patient to health.

Clinical Pearls

1. Recurrences of nonmenstrual TSS are rare, but menstrual TSS can recur in the same patient.

2. Therapy with antistaphylococcal antibiotic during the acute illness decreases the rate of recurrence.

3. Eighty percent of adults have high antibody titers to TSST-1, but 95% of patients who develop TSS have low or no antibody titers to TSST-1.

REFERENCES

1. Erstad BL, Witte CL, Talkington DF: Toxic shock-like syndrome. Pharmacotherapy 1992; 12:23–27.
2. Strausbaugh LJ: Toxic shock syndrome: Are you recognizing its changing presentations? Postgrad Med 1993; 94:107–108.
3. Fisher CJ, Celi LA: Toxic shock syndrome. In Ayres SM, Grenvik A, Holbrook PR, Shoemaker WC (eds): Textbook of Critical Care. Philadelphia, WB Saunders, 1995, pp 1305–1309.
4. Chance TD: Toxic shock syndrome: Role of the environment, the host, and the microorganism. Br J Biomed Sci 1996;53:284–289.
5. Stevens DL: The toxic shock syndromes. Infect Dis Clin North Am 1996;10:727–746.

PATIENT 76

A 25-year-old African-American woman with fever and bilateral interstitial opacities

A 25-year-old African-American woman presents to an outpatient office with a 2-month history of fevers up to 38.3°C, night sweats, increasing dyspnea on exertion, and generalized malaise. Prior to this period she was in good health and very active. She reports decreased appetite with a 15-pound weight loss. She denies headache, nausea, vomiting, and diarrhea. She has not traveled recently and denies risk factors for HIV infection. A routine PPD 1 year ago was negative.

Physical Examination: Temperature 37.6°; pulse 88; respirations 24. General: well developed, well nourished. Chest: dry rales on auscultation. CBC and serum electrolytes: normal. Alkaline phosphatase: 334 IU/L. Repeat PPD: negative at 48 hours. Chest radiograph: bilateral hilar adenopathy with diffuse reticulonodular opacities (see figure).

Question: Based on the presentation and subsequent workup, what is the most likely diagnosis?

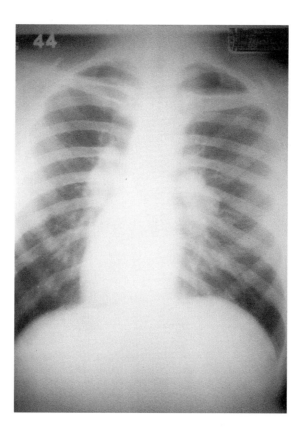

Diagnosis: Sarcoidosis

Discussion: Sarcoidosis is a multisystem, chronic, granulomatous disorder of unknown etiology that affects individuals between ages 20 and 40. The disease is more common in African-Americans than Caucasians, with a female preponderance. Most patients present with symptoms that are referable to the lung. The onset of respiratory symptoms can be acute, subacute, or chronic and may be accompanied by fatigue, malaise, anorexia, or weight loss. Some patients have cough, dyspnea, or vague retrosternal chest discomfort. Fever is present in 10% of patients, especially those with Löffgren's syndrome or liver and CNS involvement.

Sarcoidosis can present as two acute syndromes. Patients with **Löffgren's syndrome** present with erythema nodosum, uveitis with or without bilateral hilar and paratracheal adenopathy, and acute peripheral arthritis. In **Heerfordt-Waldenstrom syndrome**, patients present with fever; bilateral, nontender parotid gland enlargement (parotitis); anterior uveitis; and unilateral facial nerve palsy (Bell's palsy). Patients with sarcoidosis can have a variety of physical findings, or the physical examination may be entirely normal.

Sarcoidosis is diagnosed on routine chest radiograph in 20–40% of asymptomatic patients. Chest radiographs are abnormal in 90% of patients affected with sarcoidosis. **Bilateral hilar adenopathy**, the hallmark of sarcoidosis, is present in 97% of patients. Sarcoidosis is staged on the basis of chest radiographic findings as follows:

Stage 0   Normal chest x-ray
Stage 1   Bilateral hilar adenopathy
Stage 2   Bilateral hilar adenopathy and diffuse parenchymal opacities
Stage 3   Diffuse parenchymal opacities without hilar adenopathy
Stage 4   Lung fibrosis

Fifty percent of patients have a stage 1 chest radiograph on presentation.

Note that radiographic findings do not always correlate with the clinical presentation or disease. A computed tomography scan of the chest is useful in demonstrating parenchymal disease that is not obvious on chest radiograph. Pleural effusions are rare, but may be present in stages 2 and 3 disease.

Laboratory findings include leukemia, lymphocytopenia, elevated erythrocyte sedimentation rate and alkaline phosphatase, hypercalciuria (more common than hypercalcemia), and hypergammaglobulinemia. Serum angiotensin converting enzyme (ACE) is elevated in 40–80% of patients with acute sarcoidosis and can be used to monitor therapy and clinical progress.

The diagnosis of sarcoidosis is based on clinical, radiographic, and histologic findings. Lung diagnosis is made by mediastinoscopy or transbronchial lung biopsy with histologic findings of noncaseous or "sarcoid" granulomas and increased T-helper lymphocyte and mononuclear cell populations. Gallium scan is positive in nearly all cases, with symmetrical uptake in the parotid glands, orbits, lungs, and intrathoracic lymph nodes. Tissue biopsy supplants the need for gallium scans in most patients. Once the diagnosis of sarcoidosis is made, all patients should have an ophthalmologic examination to rule out uveitis. Steroid therapy is recommended only for symptomatic patients with: (1) symptomatic and/or deteriorating pulmonary disease, (2) hypercalcemia, and (3) extrapulmonary involvement, i.e., uveitis, cardiomyopathy, neurologic disease.

The differential diagnosis of sarcoidosis includes lymphoma, tuberculosis, malignancy, histoplasmosis, coccidioidomycosis, and brucellosis. Remission of sarcoidosis is spontaneous in acute disease, with good response to steroid therapy. These patients usually have a good prognosis. Patients who present with chronic insidious onset generally have a worse prognosis, with multiple episodes of relapsing disease. Patients with sarcoidosis may progress to endstage lung disease despite appropriate therapy.

The present patient was considered to have sarcoidosis based on an abnormal chest radiograph, elevated ACE level of 120 IU/L (normal 8–30), and positive gallium scan. She refused bronchoscopy, which was needed to confirm the diagnosis. She improved on a 6-month course of steroid therapy, with resolution of her opacities.

Organ System	Incidence (%)	Clinical Signs and Symptoms
Lungs	90	Dyspnea, chest pain, cough, parenchymal opacities ± lymphadenopathy on chest radiograph
Lymph nodes	75–90	Intrathoracic ± peripheral lymphadenopathy
Skin	25	Erythema nodosum, lupus pernio, plaques, maculopapular eruptions, subcutaneous nodules
Eyes	25	Uveitis, iritis, scleral plaques, conjunctival lesions, keratoconjunctivitis
Gastrointestinal	20	Elevated liver function tests, hepatosplenomegaly
Upper respiratory tract	10–20	Nasal granulomas, nasal stuffiness, hoarseness, wheezing, stridor
Musculoskeletal	10–20	Arthralgias, symmetric ascending polyarthritis, myopathy, erosive and cystic lesions of small bones of hands
Neurologic	5–10	Seventh nerve palsy, aseptic basilar meningitis
Salivary glands	6	Sicca syndrome, parotitis
Cardiac	5	Complete heart block, cardiac arrhythmias, sudden death

Clinical Pearls

1. Fever is rare in sarcoidosis.

2. When lymphoma, tuberculosis, and sarcoidosis are in the differential diagnosis of a patient with hilar adenopathy, a gallium scan with bilateral parotid gland uptake points to the diagnosis of sarcoidosis.

3. Lupus pernio, the most specific skin finding in sarcoidosis, suggests chronic disease.

4. Hypercalciuria is an earlier and more common finding than hypercalcemia in sarcoidosis.

REFERENCES

1. Sharma OP: Pulmonary sarcoidosis and corticosteroids. Am Rev Respir Dis 1993; 147:1598.
2. Chestnutt AN: Enigmas in sarcoidosis. West J Med 1995; 162:519–526.
3. DeRemee RA: Sarcoidosis. Mayo Clin Proc 1995; 70:177–181.

PATIENT 77

A 48-year-old woman with mitral valve prolapse, fever, petechiae, and confusion

A 48-year-old woman with a history of mitral valve prolapse presents with a 2-week history of progressive weakness, fevers to 38.8°C, and sweats. One day before presentation, her husband noted that she had some episodes of confusion and a rash on her lower extremities. The patient had a dental cleaning 6 weeks ago, at which time she was prophylaxed with erythromycin because of her allergy to penicillin. Her past medical history is significant for asthma.

Physical Examination: Temperature 38.6°; pulse 100; respirations 22; blood pressure 128/76. General: acutely ill appearance; alert and oriented to person and place, but unable to remember date. HEENT: no conjunctival petechiae, throat normal, neck supple. Chest: bibasilar rales on lung auscultation. Cardiac: grade III/VI systolic murmur at left sternal border. Abdomen: soft, nontender, no splenomegaly. Extremities: petechial rash on both lower extremities.

Laboratory Findings: WBC 16,200/μl with 86% polymorphonuclear cells, 4% bands, 8% lymphocytes, 2% monocytes; hemoglobin 10.6 mg/dl; platelets 118,000/μl; ESR 116 mm/hr. Electrolytes: normal. Urinalysis: normal. Chest radiograph: clear. Echocardiogram: moderate mitral regurgitation and small echodensity on mitral valve (see figure). Transesophageal echocardiography (TEE): ordered. Blood cultures: three sets positive for small gram-negative bacillus. CT scan of head: negative for bleeding, infarct, or abscess.

Questions: What is your diagnosis? How would you proceed?

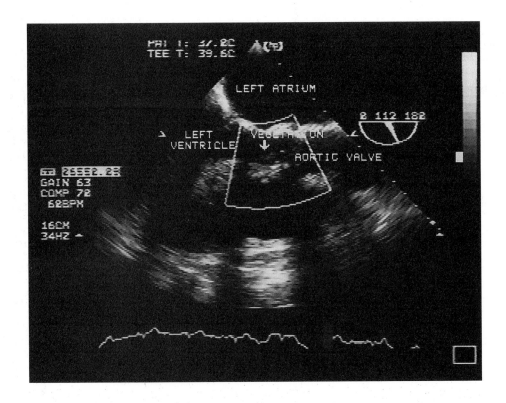

Diagnosis: Endocarditis due to *Actinobacillus actinomycetemcomitans*

Discussion: *A. actinomycetemcomitans* is a small, gram-negative, aerobic bacillus that is part of the normal oral flora. It is a rare cause of endocarditis, which occurs as a complication of periodontal disease and dental work in patients with abnormal and prosthetic valves. Endocarditis can occur after dental procedures despite prophylaxis with penicillin, erythromycin, or vancomycin. The onset of infection is insidious, with a mean time from presentation of symptoms to diagnosis of 3 months. Most patients present subacutely with fever, chills, night sweats, malaise, weight loss, and anorexia, with or without peripheral stigmata of endocarditis. Hepatomegaly and splenomegaly are common. Patients are anemic and the erythrocyte sedimentation rate is elevated almost 100% of the time. The organism is fastidious, slow growing (1–3 weeks), and difficult to culture because it requires 5–10% CO_2 for growth. Thus, the diagnosis often is delayed.

A. actinomycetemcomitans endocarditis usually is complicated by embolic events. Typical sites are the central nervous system, eye, kidney, lung, and spleen. Another complication is congestive heart failure requiring valve replacement. Death also may result. Patients who develop embolic events usually have a poor prognosis. *A. actinomycetemcomitans* can cause severe periodontal disease, especially localized juvenile periodontitis. Soft tissue infection usually occurs in association with *Actinomyces israelii* in lesions of actinomycosis. Brain and thyroid abscesses, pneumonia, empyema, pericarditis, synovitis, and osteomyelitis also can result.

The recommended therapy for endocarditis is 4–6 weeks of penicillin or ampicillin in combination with an aminoglycoside if the strain is susceptible. A cephalosporin should be used if the susceptibility of the organism to ampicillin or penicillin is questionable.

The present patient was empirically started on vancomycin and gentamicin. Blood culture results were positive for *A. actinomycetemcomitans* 1 week after admission. The TEE confirmed the presence of mitral vegetations. The patient's mental status improved, but her clinical course was complicated by worsening congestive heart failure requiring mitral valve replacement.

Clinical Pearls

1. The onset of endocarditis usually is insidious, and growth of the organism may take up to 3 weeks.

2. *A. actinomycetemcomitans* is one of the HACEK organisms (*Hemophilus aphrophilus/paraphrophilus, Cardiobacterium hominis, Eikenella corrodens,* and *Kingella kingae*), which are all slow growers in culture.

3. Soft tissue infection usually occurs in association with *Actinomyces israelii.*

REFERENCES

1. Horowitz EA, Pugsley MP, Turbes PG, et al: Pericarditis caused by *Actinobacillus actinomycetemcomitans*. J Infect Dis 1987; 155:152–153.
2. Grace CJ, Levitz RE, Katz-Pollack H, et al: *Actinobacillus actinomycetemcomitans* prosthetic valve endocarditis. Rev Infect Dis 1988; 10:922–929.
3. Kaplan AH, Weber DJ, Oddone EZ, Perfert JR: Infection due to *Actinobacillus actinomycetemcomitans:* 15 cases and review. Rev Infect Dis 1989; 11:46–63.

PATIENT 78

A 25-year-old man with fever, vesicular rash, and pneumonia

A 25-year-old man is sent to the emergency department by his family physician for evaluation of fever and vesicular rash. The patient was apparently in good health until 2 days prior to admission when he experienced a sudden onset of fever to 40°C, and a headache and nonproductive cough developed. These symptoms were followed by a maculopapular rash that progressed rapidly into vesicle formation. The rash was described as occasionally pruritic and painless and was first noted on the lower extremities. It progressed cephalad to the trunk and upper extremities, with involvement of the palms and soles.

The patient has lived all his life in New York City and reports no recent travel. He denies recent insect or animal bites, and his only exposure to animals is contact with a neighbor's cat. Currently he works as an auto mechanic. He shares an apartment with his wife and a sister who just arrived from Puerto Rico. A niece was recently ill with "a rash and fever," which resolved.

The patient had chicken pox at age 7 with no complications and received "complete" immunizations as a child. He has been sexually active only with his wife for the previous 5 years. An HIV test 1 year ago was negative.

Physical Examination: Temperature 39.6°; pulse 128; respirations 20; blood pressure 128/88. General: mildly ill. HEENT: mucous membranes intact; some carious teeth; no lymphadenopathy. Chest: occasional rhonchi in both lung fields. Cardiac: normal, tachycardic with regular rhythm, no murmurs. Abdomen: benign. Extremities: bilateral pedal edema. Skin: small (< 5 mm) vesicles on trunk, abdomen, and all four extremities, with involvement of palms and soles and some macules on the abdomen.

Laboratory Findings: Hct 44%; WBC 8400/µl with 75% neutrophils, 3% bands, 12% lymphocytes, 3% monocytes, 7% eosinophils; platelets 220,000/µl; ESR 38 mm/hr. Prothrombin time 12.3 sec (12.2 control), partial prothrombin time 30 sec (30 control). Routine chemistries: normal. Urinalysis: unremarkable. Chest radiograph: right lower lobe consolidation with mild pleural effusion (see figure). Arterial blood gas (room air): mild hypoxemia with a normal A-a gradient. Blood and urine cultures: infectious disease consult requested.

Questions: What is this patient's likely diagnosis? What antibiotic(s) or antiviral agent should be initiated? Should other tests be ordered?

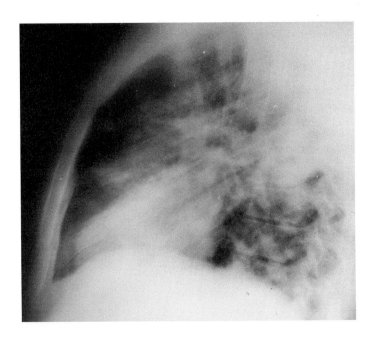

Diagnosis: Atypical measles

Discussion: Since its original description in 1965, the atypical measles syndrome has been extensively described in the literature. The diagnosis is often missed because it is not considered in the differential diagnosis or, as is more often the case, it is unfamiliar to most clinicians. Atypical measles is a clearly defined clinical syndrome that occurs predominantly in young men and women who initially received primary immunization with inactivated (killed) measles vaccine after exposure to natural measles. There have been a few reports, however, of cases among those previously immunized with the live vaccines. The killed viral vaccine was given from 1963 to 1968 and then pulled off the market because live viral vaccines became available.

After an incubation period of 1–2 weeks (similar to typical measles), patients develop a prodrome of acute onset of high fever (39.4°–40.5°C) and nonspecific complaints such as headache, nonproductive cough, myalgia, vague abdominal pain, and generalized malaise. In contrast to typical measles, coryza, conjunctivitis, and Koplik's spots are rare occurrences. Two to three days after the onset of the prodromal symptoms, a rash unlike that seen in typical measles appears on the extremities and proceeds centrifugally or cephalad. The rash characteristically is erythematous and maculopapular, usually pruritic, and may progress to vesicular lesions. Unlike the vesicular lesions of varicella, lesions do not form scabs. Occasionally the rash may have a petechial component, prompting the clinician to consider the diagnoses of Rocky Mountain spotted fever and meningococcemia in the absence of other characteristic signs and symptoms. Edema of the lower extremities also has been described.

There is a high frequency of respiratory involvement with pneumonia. Indeed, there are numerous reports of atypical measles with pneumonia and an abnormal chest radiograph as the predominant manifestations, and these patients may (rarely) present without a rash. Chest radiographs typically show consolidation, but other findings also are common, including nodules, effusions, and hilar adenopathy. Occasionally, nodules persist for months to years with no accompanying sequelae.

Laboratory findings are nonspecific, but a mild leukopenia, eosinophilia, and an elevated ESR tend to be consistent. Measles serology by CF or hemagglutination inhibition (HAI) is the most helpful laboratory test. In natural measles infection, both CF and HAI titers rarely go above 1:160, while the titers in atypical measles are usually ≥1:1024.

The prognosis is good and treatment is largely supportive. The most important goal of therapy is to identify the syndrome early so as to eliminate unnecessary, often expensive tests and avoid the use of potentially harmful antimicrobial agents. The diagnosis is made by the occurrence of the characteristic signs and symptoms in a young adult with a history of primary immunization to measles (more commonly with the killed viral vaccine), a recent exposure to natural measles infection, and elevated measles serology.

The present patient improved with "expectant management" and bed rest. Interestingly, he received the killed vaccine during childhood and the live virus vaccine as a military recruit 7 years ago.

Clinical Pearls

1. Atypical measles is a clearly defined syndrome characterized by acute onset of fever followed by a characteristic maculopapular or vesicular rash progressing centrifugally or cephalad.

2. The syndrome occurs in young adults previously immunized with measles vaccine, most frequently in recipients of the killed virus vaccine after a recent exposure to a natural measles infection.

3. A chest radiograph should be performed in all patients suspected to have atypical measles because virtually all of those affected will show opacities, nodules, effusions, or hilar adenopathy.

4. The characteristic signs and symptoms with a markedly elevated measles titer on serology (≥ 1:1024) confirm the diagnosis.

5. In the presence of a petechial rash component, Rocky Mountain spotted fever and meningococcemia must be ruled out.

REFERENCES

1. Sharpe RJ, Albert LS, Imber MJ, Haynes HA: Isolation of a viable virus from a patient with atypical measles and rash in an inverse photodistribution. J Am Acad Dermatol 1990; 22:1107–1109.
2. Nichols KJ: Atypical measles: A diagnostic conundrum. J Am Osteopath Assoc 1991; 91:691–694.
3. Cherry JD: Measles. *In* Feigin RD, Cherry JD (eds): Textbook of Pediatric Infectious Disease. 3rd ed. Philadelphia, WB Saunders Co., 1992, pp 1591–1609.
4. Wong RD, Goetz MB: Clinical and laboratory features of measles in hospitalized adults. Am J Med 1993; 95:377–383.

PATIENT 79

A 44-year-old diabetic man with diarrhea, abdominal pain, and fever

A 44-year-old man with Type I diabetes mellitus has suffered an acute onset of crampy right lower quadrant abdominal pain, diarrhea, fever, and chills. The diarrhea is severe, occurring 10–15 times a day; scant in volume; and occasionally blood-tinged. He reports eating barbecued chicken and tossed green salad at a party 2 days previously. He has reduced his insulin because he "has not been eating" since the onset of symptoms. The patient has no history of recent travel or exposure to pets and denies the presence of HIV risk factors.

Physical Examination: Temperature 38.8°; pulse 130; respirations 32; blood pressure 98/60. General: acutely ill appearance, tachypneic. HEENT: dry oral mucosa. Chest: clear to auscultation. Cardiac: S_1S_2 normal, rhythm regular, no murmurs. Abdomen: soft and diffusely tender; pain most severe in lower quadrants; no rebound tenderness; hyperactive bowel sounds. Extremities: no edema. Skin: no rash.

Laboratory Findings: WBC 15,500/µl with 84% polymorphonuclear cells, 2% bands, 14% lymphocytes; platelets 420,000/µl. Routine chemistries: serum glucose 618 mg/dl, prerenal azotemia, high anion gap metabolic acidosis. Arterial blood gas: confirms acidosis. Urine and serum ketone tests: positive. Blood, urine, and stool cultures: pending. Additional studies for fecal leukocytes, ova, and parasites: pending. Chest radiograph: normal. Abdominal radiographs: nonspecific bowel gas pattern. Direct microscopy of fecal specimen: numerous WBCs and RBCs; motile organisms (by phase contrast; see figure).

Question: What is the likely pathogen causing the diarrhea?

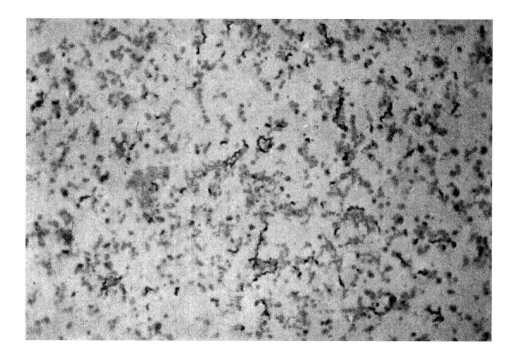

Diagnosis: *Campylobacter jejuni* infection

Discussion: Campylobacter organisms are present in the gastrointestinal tract of most animals used for food; therefore, a large proportion of the meat supply is contaminated during food processing. Infection with these organisms is common, and *Campylobacter* spp. is the most common cause of bacterial diarrhea in the United States, with *C. jejuni* as the most frequent isolate. The other species cause practically the same manifestations. It appears that poultry is the most significant source based on several studies reporting both epidemic and sporadic infections. The organisms are killed by heating, and undercooked meat or contamination of kitchen surfaces and utensils are significant sources of infection.

The incubation period is 1–7 days after ingestion of contaminated food. Enteric manifestations are usually heralded by a prodrome of flu-like illness, with fever, myalgia, headache, and body malaise, which may be accompanied by diarrhea. The diarrhea usually takes the form of loose, occasionally bloody, stools. Frequency is variable, with a few episodes of greater than 20 bowel movements per day. In one consequence of infection, colitis, the predominant manifestations are bloody stools, excessive abdominal cramping, and fever. At the extreme end of the clinical spectrum, toxic megacolon may arise. The majority of infections, however, are self-limited and seldom last beyond 1 week.

The diagnosis usually is made by a positive stool culture, although blood cultures are sometimes positive. An early presumptive diagnosis can be made by direct microscopy demonstration of fecal WBCs and RBCs and bacteria with characteristic darting motility.

Therapy is mainly supportive with replacement of lost fluids and electrolytes. Some clinicians advocate antimicrobial therapy *early* during the illness, as delayed treatment does not significantly alter the course of the disease. Thus, early diagnosis is the key. There is general agreement that patients with severe symptoms—high fever with bloody diarrhea, more than 10 loose stools per day, and symptoms persisting beyond 1 week—should be treated. Erythromycin is considered the antimicrobial therapy of choice. Effective alternative agents include the quinolones and tetracyclines. Therapy is continued for 5–7 days. Unlike infections with *Salmonella* spp., antimicrobial therapy does not prolong carriage of *Campylobacter* and, in fact, eliminates fecal carriage within 72 hours. Patients typically recover fully after infection. Recognized sequelae of *C. jejuni* infections include reactive arthritis and Reiter's syndrome, particularly in those with positive HLA-B27, and Guillain-Barré syndrome.

In the present patient, *Campylobacter jejuni* was identified on direct microscopy of fecal specimens, and he received early antimicrobial therapy in the form of oral erythromycin. Blood, urine, and stool cultures came back positive, confirming the diagnosis. The patient's diabetes had been exacerbated by the infectious diarrhea and was easily controlled after the infection was treated. He slowly recovered over the subsequent 2 weeks.

Clinical Pearls

1. *Campylobacter jejuni,* the most common cause of infectious bacterial diarrhea in the United States, is transmitted by contaminated meat or water.

2. In normal hosts bacteremia is infrequent, usually transient, and does not require therapy. Bacteremia is more common in compromised hosts, e.g., hypogammaglobulinemic individuals, and may be prolonged with resulting severe illness.

3. Symptomatic improvement results if antibiotic therapy (ideally, erythromycin) is begun within 3 days of illness. A delay in the institution of therapy beyond 4 days eliminates any benefit; therefore, early recognition and diagnosis are key factors. Erythromycin therapy at any point, however, results in the elimination of fecal carriage.

4. Demonstration of WBCs, RBCs, and bacteria with darting motility by direct microscopy of a fecal smear is sufficient for a presumptive diagnosis of *Campylobacter* diarrhea.

5. Reiter's syndrome, reactive arthritis, and Guillain-Barré syndrome are frequently recognized sequelae of *Campylobacter* infection.

REFERENCES

1. Cornick NA, Gorbach SL: *Campylobacter*. Infect Dis Clin North Am 1988; 2(3):643–654.
2. Blaser MJ: *Campylobacter* and related species. In Mandell GL, Bennett JE, Dolin R (eds): Principles and Practice of Infectious Diseases. 4th ed. New York, Churchill Livingstone, Inc., 1995, pp 1948–1956.
3. Blaser MJ: Epidemiologic and clinical features of *Campylobacter jejuni* infections. J Infect Dis 1997; 176 (Suppl 2):S103–105.

PATIENT 80

A 20-year-old Italian man with fever and pleuritis

A 20-year-old Italian man presents to the emergency department with an acute onset of left-sided chest pain. The pain is persistent, pleuritic, radiating to the ipsilateral upper shoulder, and not relieved by rest. He denies any other symptoms, but states that he had a similar, milder episode of the same symptoms 4 months ago. At that time, his chest pain was associated with a low-grade fever and vague abdominal pain. He took aspirin tablets, but relief was variable. He did not seek medical attention because the symptoms were mild, and they disappeared after 3 days. The patient was a college soccer player and has been healthy. His family history is negative for cardiovascular disease, and he denies illicit drug use.

Physical Examination: Temperature 39°; pulse 102; respirations 22; blood pressure 118/78. General: anxious but otherwise "nontoxic" appearance. HEENT: no abnormalities. Chest: no evidence of chest wall trauma, no chest wall tenderness, decreased breath sounds on left base, no rubs appreciated, no evidence of consolidation. Cardiac: S_1S_2 normal, rhythm regular, no murmurs. Abdomen: normal. Skin: no rash. Lymph nodes: no adenopathy.

Laboratory Findings: Hct 38%; WBC 19,000/μl with 90% neutrophils, 2% bands, 7% lymphocytes, 1% monocytes; platelets 280,000/μl. Routine chemistries: normal. Aspartate aminotransferase: mildly elevated. Urinalysis: normal. Routine cultures: pending. Electrocardiogram: sinus tachycardia. Chest radiograph: small left pleural effusion, normal bony structures, no opacities. Computed tomography scan of abdomen: see figure.

Question: What is your diagnosis and how would you pursue it?

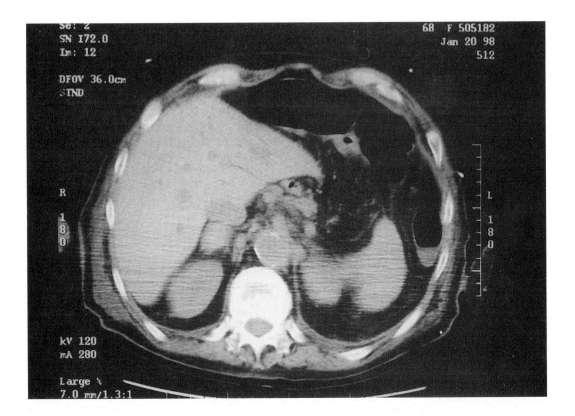

Diagnosis: Familial Mediterranean fever

Discussion: Familial Mediterranean fever (FMF) is an inherited disorder of unknown etiology, characterized by a periodic occurrence of fever, polyserositis, and arthritis. Cases occur predominantly among Sephardic Jews and those of Arabic and Armenian descent. Infrequently, FMF is seen in Ashkenazi Jews and Italians. Up to 50% of patients report a negative family history. A high degree of consanguinity also is observed.

The disease occurs early in life, usually first appearing in childhood or late adolescence. The periodic occurrence, frequency, and severity of symptoms vary among patients. Succeeding episodes may be milder or more severe, e.g., with involvement of multiple serosal structures. **Fever** is the most common manifestation and is the cardinal feature of the disorder. The fever may range from low- to high-grade. **Abdominal pain** as a result of peritonitis is the next most common feature, occurring in up to 95% of patients. Initially localized, it eventually involves the entire abdomen. Patients presenting for the first time generally undergo a laparotomy. Operative findings are normal except for a peritoneal effusion that produces normal results in routine fluid studies. Pleuritis may occur simultaneously with peritonitis. Rarely, pleuritis precedes peritonitis or is the only manifestation of serositis. Chest pain usually is unilateral, with effusions, friction rubs, or diminished breath sounds.

Arthritis in FMF occurs exclusively in children and is observed in up to 75%. Joint involvement typically is monoarticular or asymmetrical, predominantly large joints, and nonerosive. Deforming sequelae are not known to occur. Other, less common manifestations include pericarditis; meningitis; and skin lesions, which typically appear as an erythematous, circumscribed rash mimicking erysipelas. Amyloidosis occurs as a complication of FMF and is most commonly observed among patients from Israel and the Middle East. The involvement of other organ systems, resulting in (for example) splenomegaly, hematuria, and proteinuria, is more likely when amyloidosis is present.

Most of the laboratory findings in FMF during acute attacks are nonspecific, i.e., elevated ESR, serum fibrinogen, and leukocytosis. Abnormalities in urinalysis reflect amyloidosis.

Diagnosis usually is made without difficulty in a patient with the appropriate ethnic background and typical presentation. Other causes of periodic fevers to be considered during atypical attacks include hyperimmunoglobulinemia D, cyclic neutropenia, and the FAPA syndrome, which is characterized by periodic fever, aphthous ulcers, pharyngitis, and adenopathy. These conditions usually can be diagnosed by characteristic clinical and/or laboratory findings.

There is no known effective therapy for acute attacks of FMF. Treatment is supportive at best, with analgesics. Colchicine has been in use for the last two decades as prophylaxis for acute attacks, with one series reporting a 70% favorable response rate.

The present patient had nonanatomic chest pain and no cardiovascular conditions. A diagnosis of familial Mediterranean fever was made based on the patient's ancestry and the similar episode of chest pain 4 months earlier. He responded to a course of colchicine treatment.

Clinical Pearls

1. Familial Mediterranean fever should be considered in patients of appropriate ethnic background who present with periodic fevers accompanied by signs and symptoms of peritonitis, pleuritis, and monoarticular arthritis. A negative family history does not rule out FMF.

2. Splenomegaly and kidney involvement should warrant consideration of amyloidosis.

3. Colchicine is effective for prophylaxis of acute attacks of FMF.

REFERENCES

1. Zemer D, Livneh A, Danon YL, et al: Long-term colchicine treatment in children with familial Mediterranean fever. Arthritis Rheum 1991; 34:973–977.
2. Lightfoot RW, Jr: Intermittent and periodic arthritic syndromes. *In* McCarty DJ, Koopman WJ (eds): Arthritis and Allied Conditions. Philadelphia, Lea and Febiger, 1993, pp 1125–1130.
3. Livneh A, Langevitz P, Zemer D, et al: The changing face of familial Mediterranean fever. Semin Arthritis Rheum 1996; 26:612–627.
4. Kees S, Langevitz P, Zemer D, et al: Attacks of pericarditis as a manifestation of familial Mediterranean fever (FMF). QJM 1997; 90:643–647.
5. Livneh A, Langevitz P, Zemer D, et al: Criteria for the diagnosis of familial Mediterranean fever. Arthritis Rheum 1997; 40:1879–1885.

PATIENT 81

A 5-year-old girl with cellulitis of the left cheek

A 5-year-old girl was noted by her mother to be irritable and "feverish" 1 day prior to admission. The patient was rushed to the emergency department after she became lethargic and a purplish-red discoloration appeared on her left cheek. She was admitted with a diagnosis of cellulitis and was started on ceftizoxime after specimens for blood and urine cultures were collected.

Physical Examination: Temperature 40.6°. General: acutely ill appearance; irritable. HEENT: warm, tender, dark-colored cellulitic rash on left cheek; mild bulging and haziness of the left tympanic membrane. Neurologic: no localizing signs nor deficits.

Laboratory Findings: Hct 44%; WBC 19,200/μl with 73% neutrophils, 17% stabs 10% lymphocytes; platelets 485,000/μl. Routine chemistries: normal. Urinalysis: 1+ proteinuria; otherwise normal.

Questions: What is the most likely etiology of the cellulitis? Are additional evaluations or therapies needed?

Diagnosis: Type b facial cellulitis due to *Haemophilus influenzae*

Discussion: *Haemophilus influenzae* is normally found in the upper respiratory tract of most humans. The bacteria are primarily colonized by nonencapsulated strains, but up to 5% of isolates reveal capsules which are commonly serotype b. Type b strains usually cause invasive infections such as meningitis, epiglottitis, cellulitis (typically with bacteremia), and pneumonia. In fact, most *Haemophilus* invasive diseases in children are attributed to type b strains.

Acute *H. influenzae* facial cellulitis in children and infants is a serious and potentially life-threatening infection. The area usually involved is one cheek (buccal cellulitis) or the periorbital (preseptal cellulitis) area. The child's illness typically starts with rapid onset of fever $> 38.8°C$ and toxicity. Patients frequently have upper respiratory tract complaints beginning 3–7 days before onset of the acute febrile illness. A cellulitic rash immediately follows the onset of fever (within 24 hours). The rash typically has a purplish-red hue, which is a helpful diagnostic sign. Group A streptococcus, the next most common cause of facial cellulitis in this age group, characteristically presents with an erysipelas-type rash.

Buccal cellulitis is thought to arise from a local, occasionally inapparent mouth trauma which encourages invasion of the adjacent soft tissues, or from an ipsilateral otitis media which involves the soft tissue by lymphatic spread. Cases of **periorbital cellulitis** usually have an underlying ethmoid or maxillar sinusitis. In evaluating patients with buccal cellulitis the clinician should look for periorbital involvement, which may occur concurrently and be subtle on initial examination. Periorbital cellulitis must be differentiated from intraorbital infection with secondary periorbital cellulitis, as this latter condition can have disastrous consequences if left untreated (or inadequately treated). Therefore, the workup for periorbital cellulitis always should include a CT scan to make this distinction.

Initial laboratory findings show only nonspecific findings of leukocytosis. Blood cultures are positive in 75% of cases; in these patients, the bacteremia gives rise to the cellulitis and not the other way around. Needle aspiration of the margin of the cellulitis area, though rarely indicated, yields the organism on Gram stain or culture in most cases. Other, distant sites also may be involved, and meningitis occurs concomitantly in 10–20% of cases of acute bacteremic facial cellulitis. Most experts recommend performing a lumbar puncture even in patients without a clinically apparent meningitis, to give antibiotic doses adequate for penetration of the central nervous system and corticosteroids if the cerebrospinal fluid suggests a concomitant meningitis.

The preferred antimicrobial agent is a third-generation cephalosporin given intravenously. Ceftizoxime, cefotaxime, and ceftriaxone are all acceptable. Increasing reports of resistance have put ampicillin out of favor. In general, the choice of agent should take into consideration activity against *H. influenzae* and ability to cross the blood-brain barrier in the event of concomitant meningitis. Therapy for cellulitis should continue for 1–2 weeks. Additionally, all patients should receive rifampin prior to or at time of discharge, as the initial treatment course does not reliably eradicate nasopharyngeal carriage of the organism. Rifampin prophylaxis also should be given to all household contacts when the patient is < 4 years old and to all adults (contraindicated in pregnant women) in the household who have contact with susceptible children < 4 years old.

With the widespread use of *H. influenzae* type b (Hib) conjugate vaccines in the United States since 1988, the incidence of invasive disease due to this pathogen has decreased by almost 95%. Interestingly, our patient did not receive Hib vaccine as part of her immunization schedule. If there was a reason, it is unknown.

In the present patient, blood cultures were positive for *H. influenzae* type b, which is not uncommon in children and in elderly patients with chronic obstructive pulmonary disease. The presence of a purplish-red rash confirmed the diagnosis. She was treated successfully with ceftizoxime and made an uneventful recovery.

Clinical Pearls

1. Cellulitis is accompanied by bacteremia in 75% patients. Typically, buccal cellulitis arises from local (sometimes inapparent) mouth trauma or otitis media, and periorbital (preseptal) cellulitis arises from ethmoid or maxillary sinusitis.

2. The presence of a purplish-red, cellulitic rash is a helpful diagnostic clue that distinguishes the disorder from Group A streptococcal cellulitis.

3. *H. influenzae* type b facial cellulitis with bacteremia usually is accompanied by a concomitant, often clinically inapparent meningitis, especially in children.

4. All patients treated for invasive infections due to *H. influenzae* type b should receive rifampin prophylaxis prior to or at time of discharge to eliminate the nasopharyngeal carriage state.

REFERENCES

1. Halperin SA: Haemophilus influenzae type b and its role in diseases of the head and neck. J Otolaryngol 1990; 19:169–174.
2. Janai H, Stutman HR, Marks MI: Invasive *Haemophilus influenzae* type b infections: A continuing challenge. Am J Infect Control 1990; 18(3):160–166.
3. Stanley TV, Jogose M: *Haemophilus influenzae* type b cellulitis. New Zealand Med J 1991; 104(971):334–336.
4. Murphy TF: Haemophilus. In Gorbach SL, Bartlett JG, Blacklow NR (eds): Infectious Diseases. Philadelphia, W. B. Saunders Co., 1992, pp 1521–1531.
5. Centers for Disease Control and Prevention: Progress toward elimination of *Haemophilus influenzae* type b disease among infants and children—United States, 1987–1993. JAMA 1994; 271(16):1231–1232.
6. Schwartz GR, Wright SW: Changing bacteriology of periorbital cellulitis. Ann Intern Med 1996; 28:617–620.

PATIENT 82

A 28-year-old man with acquired immunodeficiency syndrome, cough, weight loss, and bilateral opacities

A 28-year-old man presents in the emergency department with complaints of fever, minimally productive cough, and 20-pound weight loss over a 3-week period. He is an intravenous drug user, and he was diagnosed with AIDS 5 months previously after presenting with *Pneumocystis carinii* pneumonia. The patient reports a maximum temperature of 39.4°C, increasing dyspnea, and blood-tinged sputum 2 days prior to admission. His last CD_4 count, obtained during the previous hospitalization, was 175/µl; at that time he refused antiretroviral therapy. He has since been lost to follow-up. The patient stopped taking trimethoprim-sulfamethoxazole for prophylaxis against *P. carinii* pneumonia 3 months ago. He admittedly has not stopped using intravenous heroin. The patient is a native of Puerto Rico. Except for a short stay in the islands 3 months previously, he has lived in New York City for the last 15 years.

Physical Examination: Temperature 39.4°; pulse 128; respirations 26; blood pressure 108/60. General: ill appearing. HEENT: pale conjunctivae, no oropharyngeal ulcers, no thrush. Chest: coarse rales bilaterally. Cardiac: S_1S_2 normal; regular rhythm; 3/6 systolic ejection murmur. Abdomen: no tenderness; palpable liver edge 3 cm below right costal margin, smooth edge. Extremities: no clubbing, no Janeway lesions, no Osler's nodes. Skin: erythematous maculopapular rash over the abdomen, back, and extremities predominantly on extensor surfaces. Lymph nodes: bilateral, small axillary and inguinal lymphadenopathies.

Laboratory Findings: Hct 28%; WBC 3800/µl with 76% neutrophils, 4% bands, 15% lymphocytes, 5% monocytes; platelets 48,000/µl. PT and PTT: normal. Aspartate aminotransferase 111 IU/L, alanine aminotransferase 98 IU/L, alkaline phosphatase 233 IU/L, total bilirubin 2.1, albumin 2.8, cholesterol 114 mg/dl, LDH 338 IU/L. Urinalysis: 2+ proteinuria, otherwise normal. Arterial blood gas: respiratory alkalosis with mild hypoxemia. Chest radiograph: bilateral interstitial opacities (worse in comparison to previous films), with some alveolar opacities predominantly in the upper lobes (see figure). Routine bacterial cultures: pending. Acid-fast bacillus study: pending.

Questions: What is the pathogen responsible for this patient's illness? What is your diagnosis?

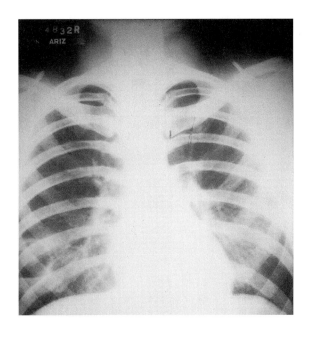

Diagnosis: Acute disseminated histoplasmosis

Discussion: Progressive disseminated histoplasmosis (PDH) encompasses a clinical spectrum which in its severe form (acute PDH) presents with a fulminant course resembling septic shock. At the other end of the spectrum is chronic PDH, with mild symptoms usually referable to a specific organ system, mainly the upper gastrointestinal tract. Subacute PDH presents with more, usually nonspecific symptoms than chronic PDH and progresses to acute PDH if left untreated. Acute PDH traditionally occurs in young children and other patients with various forms of cell-mediated immune defect. The AIDS epidemic has contributed to increased reports in the medical literature: PDH is a common first manifestation of AIDS and is a major manifestation among patients from endemic areas. PDH plus AIDS even is reported among patients in areas considered nonendemic for *Histoplasma capsulatum,* which represents reactivated disease. AIDS and other opportunistic infections become apparent with the onset of PDH, usually when the CD_4 count is $< 200/\mu l$.

The most common symptoms of acute PDH are fever, weight loss, malaise, cough, and dyspnea. Lymphadenopathy is prominent, although its value in the diagnosis is uncertain because of the frequent finding of lymphadenopathy in HIV-infected individuals. Hepatosplenomegaly is seen in up to 30% of patients. Cutaneous lesions occur in approximately 10% of patients (rare in other forms of PDH) and can appear anywhere as maculopapular eruptions. The central nervous system frequently is involved, manifesting as meningitis. Oropharyngeal ulcers are uncommon in acute PDH, contrasting with their status as the predominant manifestation in chronic PDH.

Leukopenia, anemia, and thrombocytopenia are the most common laboratory abnormalities. Elevated liver function tests also are typical. Abnormalities specific to other organ system involvement may be seen. The chest radiograph shows abnormalities in the majority of patients, with bilateral interstitial/reticulonodular opacities the most common findings. A fulminant course with septic shock, disseminated intravascular coagulation, respiratory failure with acute respiratory distress syndrome, and multiorgan failure frequently occurs in AIDS patients with acute PDH.

The diagnosis is made by biopsy or culture demonstration of the organism. Bone marrow biopsy with culture is the diagnostic procedure that gives the highest yield. Sputum smears and cultures initially may be negative, but the yield is increased by bronchoscopy with biopsy. Positive blood cultures are the rule, and shorter incubation times can be obtained by using the lysis centrifugation technique. Serologies are used only in rare instances when the diagnosis is unclear by tissue or culture methods.

The treatment for acute PDH in AIDS should be initiated immediately: amphotericin B at a dose of 0.6 mg/kg/day for 1 week, followed by 0.8 mg/kg three times a week to a total dose of 10–15 mg/kg, followed by suppressive therapy with 50 mg weekly. An alternative for suppressive therapy is itraconazole, 200 mg orally daily.

The present patient was admitted with the diagnosis of *Pneumocystis carinii* pneumonia (PCP). Pulmonary tuberculosis was to be ruled out. Therapy with TMP-SMX was initiated, and a bronchoscopy with bronchoalveolar lavage and biopsy was performed. Acid-fast bacilli were not demonstrated, and the silver stain was negative for PCP. On the 2nd hospital day, hypotension and worsening renal function developed, and his respiratory status deteriorated to the point that endotracheal intubation and mechanical ventilation were required. At this time, the chest radiograph showed worsening opacities with acute respiratory distress syndrome. The patient was started on ceftriaxone and erythromycin empirically. Initial cultures from the blood, urine, and sputum showed no growth. Lung biopsy specimens demonstrated *Histoplasma capsulatum,* and the same pathogen grew on the blood cultures on the 4th day of incubation. The patient was successfully treated with itraconazole.

Clinical Pearls

1. In AIDS patients, acute PDH may occur concurrently with other opportunistic infections. In PDH with subtle manifestations or in early PDH, the diagnosis may be missed or attributed incorrectly.

2. Acute PDH affects mostly young children and adults with cell-mediated immune defects and manifests as unrelenting, high-grade fever; pancytopenia; and hepatosplenomegaly. Its course may be fulminant in AIDS patients.

3. Features that distinguish the acute form of PDH from other forms are pancytopenia, hepatosplenomegaly, skin rash, and the absence of oropharyngeal ulcers.

4. The diagnosis is made by demonstration of a histologically compatible intracellular organism or a positive culture of blood or tissue.

5. Life-long suppressive therapy is necessary in AIDS patients to prevent relapse.

REFERENCES

1. Johnson PC, Hamill RJ, Sarosi GA: Clinical review: Progressive disseminated histoplasmosis in the AIDS patient. Semin Respir Infect 1989; 4(2):139–146.
2. Ankobiah WA, Vaidya K, Powell S, et al. Disseminated histoplasmosis in AIDS. Clinicopathologic features in seven patients from non-endemic area. NY State J Med 1990;90(5):234–8.
3. Wheat LJ, Connolly-Stringfield PA, Baker RL, et al: Disseminated histoplasmosis in the acquired immune deficiency syndrome: Clinical findings, diagnosis and treatment, and review of the literature. Medicine 1990; 69(6):361–374.

PATIENT 83

A 22-year-old bisexual man with headache and flu-like syndrome

A 22-year-old college student presents to the emergency department with complaints of a subacute onset of sore throat, worsening headache, myalgia, and fever. Symptoms progressed over 3 weeks despite intake of acetaminophen. He was seen in his college clinic 10 days before and was told that he has a viral syndrome. The only notable finding at that time was oral thrush, for which he was prescribed clotrimazole troche (10 mg) five times a day for 2 weeks. He was advised to undergo an HIV test because he admitted to being bisexual and engaging in unprotected sex. The patient reports the onset of a truncal maculopapular rash and transient arthralgias 5 days previously; the rash has resolved. He generally enjoys good health. His mother and two sisters suffer from migraine headaches. He denies illicit drug use.

Physical Examination: Temperature 39°; pulse 118; respirations 118; blood pressure 110/74. General: only mildly ill appearance. HEENT: no conjunctival injection, ear discharge, or thrush; nonexudative tonsillopharyngeal congestion. Chest: clear to auscultation, no adventitious sounds. Cardiac: S_1S_2 normal, regular rhythm, no murmurs. Abdomen: nontender; liver edge palpable 3 cm below the right costal margin, liver span 11 cm, splenomegaly. Skin: no rash. Nodes: small, nontender, nonmatted anterior/posterior cervical and occipital lymphadenopathies. Neurologic: oriented to time, place, and person; meningeal signs; no deficits or other focal findings.

Laboratory Findings: Hct 45%; WBC 11,500/μl with 93% neutrophils, 3% lymphocytes, 1% monocytes, 3% atypical lymphocytes; platelets 210,000/μl. Routine chemistries: normal except aspartate aminotransferase 51 IU/L, alanine aminotransferase 48 IU/L, alkaline phosphatase 207 IU/L. ESR 45 mm/hr, heterophil-antibody test negative. Serum RPR: negative. Urinalysis: normal. Chest radiograph: normal. HIV test (performed 10 days earlier): negative. Lumbar puncture: no organisms on Gram stain; negative India ink; glucose 60 mg/dl; total protein 55 mg/dl; WBC 22/μl with differential count of 95% lymphocytes and 5% polymorphonuclear cells. Venereal Disease Research Laboratory test: negative. MRI scan of head: see figure.

Questions: What is your diagnosis? How would you proceed with your evaluation?

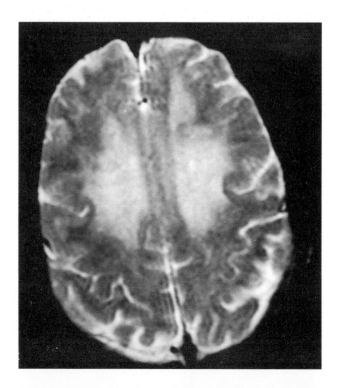

Diagnosis: HIV aseptic meningitis

Discussion: A mononucleosis-like syndrome occurs in approximately two-thirds of individuals recently infected with HIV. This phenomenon is well-described in the literature and is referred to as the acute retroviral syndrome. Symptom onset usually occurs 1–6 weeks after exposure to the virus. About one-third of patients with this syndrome present with aseptic meningitis as the predominant manifestation. Symptoms wax and wane in these patients. The prominent physical findings include lymphadenopathy which may be generalized, headache, meningismus, myalgia, arthralgias, fever, and truncal exanthem. Less common manifestations include hepatosplenomegaly, oral aphthous ulcers, and oral thrush. The rest of the physical examination is unremarkable.

Laboratory findings of patients with the acute retroviral syndrome typically reveal nonspecific abnormalities. The complete blood count may show reduced total lymphocytes, and atypical lymphocytosis may be observed. The serum transaminases and alkaline phosphatase are mildly elevated. In patients presenting with aseptic meningitis, the cerebrospinal fluid (CSF) shows a pleocytosis with a lymphocytic predominance, usually normal or mildly elevated protein, and normal glucose. The ELISA HIV test is normal in these patients, although those with an unusually prolonged illness may have positive antibodies by Western blot. Diagnosis is made by retesting the patient's serum for HIV in 3–6 months to document seroconversion. The definitive diagnosis of HIV aseptic meningitis during the acute retroviral syndrome is made by CSF viral culture or demonstration of HIV core (p24) antigen in the CSF. These procedures are not routinely performed.

Note that patients with HIV may suffer meningitis and demonstrate abnormal CSF findings in the form of lymphocytic pleocytosis at any stage of their illness. This CSF finding frequently is encountered even in asymptomatic individuals with HIV; therefore, its interpretation should take into consideration the stage of the HIV disease. Meningitis during primary HIV infection (acute seroconversion) results in prominent lymphocytic pleocytosis, normal or mildly elevated protein, and normal glucose. These findings in concert with the typical features of acute retroviral syndrome help establish the diagnosis. Approximately 50% of patients with known early HIV disease have lymphocytic pleocytosis and elevated protein levels in the CSF. As a rule, pleocytosis diminishes and protein elevation persists as HIV disease advances. The finding of lymphocytic pleocytosis in advanced HIV disease warrants exclusion of other etiologies, e.g., cryptococcus and tuberculosis, before ascribing the abnormal CSF findings to HIV.

The current patient presented with a viral prodrome that initially suggested a mononucleosis-like illness, but the thrush he experienced 10 days earlier is not a feature of a viral syndrome. During his hospital course he became encephalopathic. A computed tomography/MRI scan revealed no mass lesions, but showed white matter atrophy diagnostic of primary HIV infection of the central nervous system. The patient was treated with a variety of antiviral agents, but he died of severe dementia 9 months later.

Clinical Pearls

1. Aseptic meningitis is a common manifestation of primary HIV infection and also occurs during any stage of HIV disease.

2. As a rule, patients with early HIV disease have a lymphocytic pleocytosis, with normal to mildly elevated protein and normal glucose. Those with late disease are less likely to have pleocytosis, but mild to moderate elevations of protein may persist.

3. In attributing aseptic meningitis to HIV, syphilis should first be ruled out during early disease. In late disease with a prominent lymphocytic pleocytosis in the CSF, the following etiologies should be ruled out: *Cryptococcus neoformans, Histoplasma capsulatum, Coccidioides immitis, Mycobacterium tuberculosis, Herpes simplex* 1 and 2, lymphoma, and parameningeal processes.

REFERENCES

1. Hollander H, Stringari S: Human immunodeficiency virus-associated meningitis: Clinical course and correlations. Am J Med 1987; 83(5):813–816.
2. Denning DW: The neurological features of acute HIV infection. Biomed Pharmacother 1988; 42(1):11–14.
3. Connolly K, Hammer SM: The acute aseptic meningitis syndrome. Infect Dis Clin North Am 1990; 4:599–622.
4. Hollander H: Neurologic and psychiatric manifestations of HIV disease. J General Int Med 1991; 6(1 Suppl):S24–31.
5. Brew BJ, Currie JN: HIV-related neurological disease. Med J Australia 1993; 158(2):104–108.
6. Nelsen S, Sealy DP, Schneider EF: The aseptic meningitis syndrome. Amer Fam Phys 1993; 48:809–815.
7. Harrison MS, Simonte SJ, Kauffman CA: Trimethoprim-induced aseptic meningitis in a patient with AIDS. Clin Infect Dis 1994; 19:431–434.

PATIENT 84

A 24-year-old pregnant woman with fever, dry cough, and pancytopenia

A 24-year-old woman in her 30th week of gestation (G1P0) complains of fever and nonproductive cough of 6-week duration. Except for mild dyspnea on exertion, she reports no other symptoms. The patient illegally entered the United States from El Salvador with her husband 2 years earlier. She was a farm worker there, and she has been working off and on in the United States as a migrant farm worker. She denies ever having been sick in the past. She stopped working when she learned of her pregnancy, but she has not seen an obstetrician. Her husband also is a migrant farm worker; he worked as a hospital aide in El Salvador.

Physical Examination: Temperature 39.6°; pulse 118; respirations 24; blood pressure 100/64. HEENT: pale conjunctivae, nonicteric sclerae, small posterior cervical nodes. Chest: decreased breath sounds on both bases, crackles on both upper lung fields. Cardiac: S_1S_2 normal, regular rhythm, 2/6 systolic ejection murmur at left sternal border. Abdomen: uterine fundus height appropriate to gestational age, fetal heart sounds 145 bpm at right lower quadrant. Extremities: 2 + pitting edema of the lower extremities. Skin: no rash.

Laboratory Findings: Hct 31%; WBC 6600/μl with 60% polymorphonuclear cells, 12% bands, 18% lymphocytes, 18% atypical lymphocytes, 6% monocytes; platelets 85,000/μl. Routine chemistries: aspartate aminotransferase 58 IU/L, alanine aminotransferase 53 IU/L, alkaline phosphatase 183 IU/L, bilirubin 1.3 mg/dl, lactate dehydrogenase 202 IU/L, globulin 6.6 g/dl, albumin 2.1 g/dl. Urinalysis: normal. Chest radiograph: multiple, bilateral, punctate opacities.

Questions: What additional diagnostic tests should be performed? What treatment should be initiated?

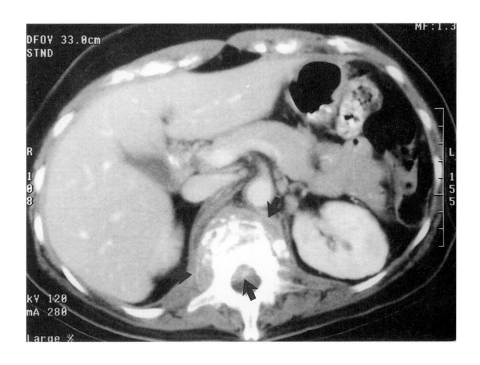

Diagnosis: Miliary tuberculosis

Discussion: Miliary tuberculosis is the term used for all forms of tuberculosis arising from widespread hematogenous dissemination of *Mycobacterium tuberculosis,* which results in tiny foci distributed primarily in the lungs and other viscera. Frequently, the lungs appear normal radiographically. The presentation typically is variable, leading to diagnostic difficulties. Although overlap may occur, miliary tuberculosis can be grouped clinicopathologically: (1) **acute miliary tuberculosis** features a prompt and typical tissue reaction to the bacilli, with few or absent bacilli demonstrable in smears; (2) **cryptic miliary tuberculosis** results in a longer disease course, often with a diminished histopathologic response, i.e., minimal granuloma formation; and (3) **nonreactive tuberculosis** causes minimal or absent organized tissue response, but a significant number of bacilli are evident histologically, and there is a septic clinical symptomatology.

Groups that show increased frequency of miliary tuberculosis include ethnic minorities; those in immunosuppressed states or using immunosuppressive agents; those with underlying medical illnesses such as alcoholism, cirrhosis, malignancies; and pregnant women. Symptoms are nonspecific and usually consist of fever, weight loss, sweats, dry cough, and malaise. Local symptoms, such as headache in meningitis or abdominal pain in peritonitis, may offer some diagnostic value. Physical examination typically reveals nonspecific findings. Clues to the diagnosis frequently are provided by peculiarities such as unusual skin eruptions, sinus tracts, and enlarged nodes; biopsies of these findings may show the characteristic pathologic features and/or the pathogen.

The diagnosis of miliary tuberculosis requires isolation of the organism from clinical specimens. However, isolation and growth are time-consuming, limiting this method's utility in critically ill patients. In these patients, less sensitive and less specific procedures such as acid-fast bacillus (AFB) stains and biopsies may be relied upon to arrive at a diagnosis and allow initiation of specific antitubercular therapy. An anergic response to purified protein derivative (PPD) and other skin tests occurs frequently in miliary tuberculosis; therefore, caution should be used in interpreting negative results. Diagnostic tests resulting in a high diagnostic yield are bronchoscopy with biopsy, liver biopsy, and bone marrow aspiration and biopsy; specimens also are sent for culture and sensitivity studies. In a patient with hematologic abnormalities, the diagnostic yield of bone marrow aspiration and biopsy approaches

100%. Liver biopsy also results in a high diagnostic yield, but is a much more invasive procedure.

The general guidelines for therapy of miliary tuberculosis during pregnancy are essentially the same as for nonpregnant patients. Initial therapy consists of isoniazid and rifampin (both pregnancy category C classification). Ethambutol is relatively safe during pregnancy and may be used until sensitivity results are obtained, to avoid the potential for isoniazid resistance. Vitamin B6 should be added to the regimen. Streptomycin should be avoided because of the risk of fetal eighth cranial nerve damage. There is not enough data to assess the safety of pyrazinamide during pregnancy; therefore, its use should be reserved for crisis situations, such as the presence of resistant organisms or adverse reactions to other first-line agents. Therapy is continued for at least 1 year.

There is a long-standing controversy regarding the effect of pregnancy on tuberculosis and tuberculosis on pregnancy. A review of the literature supports the observation that pregnancy does not adversely affect the activity of *M. tuberculosis* and vice-versa. The previously held view of therapeutic abortion was abandoned, long ago. In general, a good response to chemotherapy is achieved if used promptly and appropriately. Mothers taking antitubercular drugs can breastfeed their infants with no risks.

The present patient was admitted to a local hospital with a diagnosis of pneumonia. After appropriate cultures were obtained, she was started on ceftriaxone and erythromycin. Her hospital course worsened, with increasing dyspnea, unremitting fever, and worsening pulmonary opacities. She was transferred to a university medical center on the third hospital day. At this time, the antibiotics were changed to piperacillin, ceftazidime, and erythromycin. Serial complete blood counts showed steady declines. During the 5th hospital day values were: Hct 26%; WBC 2800/µl; polymorphonuclear cells 58%, bands 9%, lymphocytes 23%, atypical lymphocytes 4%, monocytes 6%; platelets 45,000/µl. Repeat liver function tests revealed increasing transaminases. Bronchoscopy was performed, but bronchoalveolar lavage specimens were negative for AFB and other pathogens. Sputum, urine, and blood cultures remained negative after 5 days. Serial-induced sputum smears for AFB, a PPD test, skin tests for candida and mumps, and an HIV test were all negative.

In light of persistent fever, pulmonary opacities, and worsening pancytopenia and liver function tests, a bone marrow needle biopsy was performed. Empiric antitubercular therapy was initiated with isoniazid, rifampin, and ethambutol. Examination of the bone marrow revealed few granulomas but no stainable organisms. The patient's symptoms showed improvement on the 5th day of antitubercular therapy, and she was afebrile by the 13th day. Bone marrow specimen cultures grew *Mycobacterium tuberculosis* after 5 weeks of incubation.

Clinical Pearls

1. Symptoms of miliary tuberculosis are nonspecific. The diagnosis mainly rests in the demonstration of the organism and/or the characteristic tissue reaction to tuberculosis in clinical specimens.

2. The liver, spleen, bone marrow, and lungs are almost uniformly involved in miliary tuberculosis, and biopsies of these sites usually are diagnostic. In patients with hematologic abnormalities, bone marrow aspiration and biopsy is the least invasive diagnostic procedure that provides the highest yield.

3. The PPD test is less frequently positive in miliary tuberculosis compared to other forms of the disease.

REFERENCES

1. Alvarez S, McCabe WR: Extrapulmonary tuberculosis revisited: A review of experience at Boston City and other hospitals. Medicine 1984; 63(1): 25–55.
2. Snider D: Pregnancy and tuberculosis. Chest 1984; 86(3 Suppl):10S–13S.
3. Kinoshita M, Ichikawa Y, Koga H, et. al: Re-evaluation of bone marrow aspiration in the diagnosis of miliary tuberculosis. Chest 1994; 106:690–692.
4. Sharma SK, Mohan A, Pande JN, et. al: Clinical profile, laboratory characteristics and outcome in miliary tuberculosis. Q J Med 1995; 88:29–37.

PATIENT 85

A 65-year-old man with fever, weight loss, and back pain

A 65-year-old man, a lifelong resident of New York City, is admitted with complaints of increasingly severe back pain, weight loss, and fever. Eight months earlier he sustained a fall while taking a shower. He reported mild, intermittent mid-back pain, but dismissed the symptom because it was infrequent. One month before admission, the pain became more persistent and gradually increased in intensity. He also noted a 20-pound weight loss over the previous 3 months and low-grade fever (high of 38°C) during the last 2 weeks. He generally enjoys good health, has been married to the same woman for 40 years, has four healthy children, and denies risk factors for HIV. He used to work as a radiology technician in a major city hospital. The patient states that a purified protein derivative (PPD) test was positive during a pre-employment physical 18 years ago.

Physical Examination: Temperature 37.8°; pulse 88; respirations 16; blood pressure 134/90. General: well appearing. HEENT: pink conjunctivae, no throat congestion, small posterior cervical lymphadenopathy. Chest: clear to auscultation, decreased breath sounds on right upper lung field. Cardiac: S_1S_2 normal, regular rhythm, no murmurs. Abdomen: normal. Back: marked tenderness localized to T10 and T11 vertebral bodies; no evident soft tissue swelling. Extremities: no edema. Skin: no rash. Neurologic: no localizing signs, no deficits.

Laboratory Findings: Hct 38%; WBC 9400/µl with 72% neutrophils, 24% lymphocytes, 4% monocytes; platelets 205,000/µl. Routine chemistries: lactate dehydrogenase 298 IU/L. ESR: 69 mm/hr. Urinalysis: normal. Chest radiograph: right upper lobe and apical scarring. Chest CT Scan: destruction and collapse of vertebral bodies T10 and T11; narrowed intervertebral disk space; T9 lytic lesions; evidence of paraspinal soft tissue swelling (see figure). PPD: 16 mm induration at 48 hours.

Questions: What is the most likely etiology of the vertebral lesions? Are additional tests necessary?

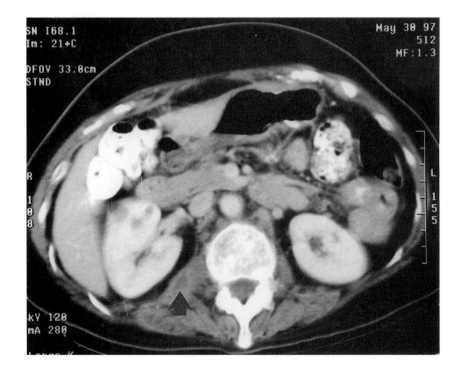

Diagnosis: Tuberculosis of the spine (tuberculous spondylitis or Pott's disease)

Discussion: Skeletal tuberculosis (TB) represents approximately 10% of all cases of extrapulmonary TB. Tuberculous osteomyelitis and arthritis of the vertebrae (spondylitis) are the most common forms of skeletal TB, occurring in 50–60% of cases. In developing countries with high rates of skeletal TB, the incidence of tuberculous spondylitis is greater in children and young adults. In developed countries, the incidence of skeletal TB has declined over the last 40 years. In this population group, the disorder is observed most frequently in middle-aged and older individuals. The advent of human immunodeficiency virus (HIV) did not appear to affect the incidence rate of skeletal TB/tuberculous spondylitis in either both developed or underdeveloped countries.

Tuberculous spondylitis is presumed to arise by reactivation of foci of infection seeded during the initial bacillemia, or by spread from the paravertebral lymph nodes. The latter observation is supported by the frequent localization of spinal TB in the thoracic vertebrae.

The patient with tuberculous spondylitis usually presents with localized pain in the back. Weight loss occurs in approximately 50%. Fever, night sweats, and anorexia occur less frequently (< 30%). Interestingly, up to 25% of patients report an antecedent trauma, thinking that their back pains are related to injury rather than to infection. In more advanced disease, a paraspinal soft tissue swelling may be evident on physical examination. Often the symptoms are so subtle that patients delay seeing a physician until symptoms of spinal cord compression supervene. *Delay in diagnosis and treatment can be catastrophic in spinal TB.*

The initial diagnostic procedure is plain radiographs of the spine. TB of the spine characteristically shows destruction of vertebral end plates, narrowing of joint space, and involvement of the intervertebral disk and the two adjacent vertebrae. With severe disk destruction, vertebral body collapse with anterior wedging results, giving rise to a "gibbus" or bump—a characteristic feature of tuberculous spondylitis. Often, paravertebral and psoas abscesses are apparent. Computed tomography scan or magnetic resonance imaging may show the bony abnormalities if plain films do not (usually

in early disease). Bone and gallium scans have a low diagnostic yield, but may be necessary to detect other unsuspected sites.

Skeletal TB may be evident alone or in conjunction with other manifestations of the disease, particularly lung disorders. Therefore, the diagnosis should be readily considered in patients with known TB. The diagnosis also is suggested in those at high risk for TB in the presence of a positive PPD and skeletal radiographic abnormalities of localized spondylitis. Confirmation is achieved by aspiration of joint fluid or soft tissue abscess, or biopsy of the bone or synovium with additional specimens sent for cultures. AFB stain of synovial fluid has a sensitivity approaching only 25%. Cultures for *Mycobacterium tuberculosis* are positive in two-thirds of cases. Biopsy greatly improves the diagnostic yield.

The differential diagnosis of tuberculous spondylitis includes brucellosis (may be clinically and radiographically indistinguishable from TB), spondylitis from other mycobacterial species, osteomyelitis with other pyogenic organisms, fungal infection, actinomycosis, lymphoma, metastatic cancer, and multiple myeloma.

Complications of tuberculous spondylitis are potentially life-threatening, e.g., paraplegia due to cord compression, meningitis due to rupture through dura, transverse myelitis, and formation of cold abscesses. Early diagnosis and therapy (medical and/or surgical) are the cornerstones, of successful intervention. Standard chemotherapy with isoniazid and rifampin usually results in a favorable outcome. For resistant strains, treatment is with four drugs for a total of 1–2 years. Most experts feel that early surgical intervention to drain bone abscesses or remove necrotic debris is necessary to achieve cure. Patients with extensive bone destruction and with neurologic findings warrant emergent surgical consultation.

The present patient was diagnosed with Pott's disease of the spine by culture of *Mycobacterium tuberculosis* from bone biopsy of the involved vertebral bodies. He was treated with antitubercular drugs, which prevented the disease from progressing but did not reverse the already destroyed vertebral bodies. The soft tissue swelling resolved with treatment.

Clinical Pearls

1. Skeletal tuberculosis is the second most common extrapulmonary form of tuberculosis next to lymphadenitis. Tuberculosis of the spine/tuberculous spondylitis is the most frequent form, occurring in up to 60% of cases.

2. The most common presenting complaint is localized back pain, followed by weight loss. Other constitutional complaints, such as fever and night sweats, or symptoms to suggest tuberculosis from other sites are less frequent.

3. The diagnosis usually is apparent in plain radiographic studies by the appearance of characteristic lesions in a patient at high-risk for tuberculosis. Therapy should not be delayed pending bacteriologic identification or biopsy results.

4. Response to standard antituberculous chemotherapy usually is good. However, surgical intervention, i.e., drainage of debris or focal abscess, may be necessary to achieve cure.

5. All patients with advanced bony destruction and/or neurologic deficits warrant immediate surgical evaluation and intervention.

REFERENCES

1. Bassam O, Robertson JM, Nelson RJ, Chin LC: Pott's disease: A resurgent challenge to the thoracic surgeon. Chest 1989; 95(1):145–150.
2. Rezai AR, Lee M, Cooper PR, et al: Modern management of spinal tuberculosis. Neurosurgery 1995;36:87–97.
3. Okuyama Y, Nakaoka Y, Kimoto K, Ozasa K: Tuberculous spondylitis (Pott's disease) with bilateral pleural effusion. Intern Med 1996; 35:883–885.
4. Parmar M, Appleton PJ: Pott's disease of the spine. Brit J Hosp Med 1996; 56:52.

INDEX

Bilirubin, serum levels of
  in hepatitis, 41, 42
  in malaria, 136, 137
Bites
  dog, as *Pasteurella multocida* infection cause, **58–59**
  insect, as streptococcal cellulitis cause, 80–81
Blood products, parvovirus B19 transmission in, 65
Bone biopsy, of chronic osteomyelitis, 96
Borrelia burgdorferi, 119, 153
Boston exanthema, 55
Botryomycosis, 74
Bradycardia, relative
  drug fever-related, 117
  legionnaire's disease-related, 148
  psittacosis-related, 121
  salmonellosis-related, 127
Bronchiectasis, 113
Brucella infections, 180
  endocarditis, 83, 84

Campylobacter jejuni infection, **187–189**
Candidiasis
  disseminated, **110–111**
  as endocarditis cause, **49–50,** 150
  hepatosplenic, **129–131**
  as prosthetic valve endocarditis cause, 150
Cardiobacterium infections, 83
Cardiovascular disease. *See also* Endocarditis
  Kawasaki disease-related, 166
Catheters, chronic ambulatory peritoneal, 158
Ceftriaxone
  as chancroid treatment, 48
  as gonorrhea treatment, 4, 14
Cellulitis
  differentiated from Sweet's syndrome, 132
  facial, **192–194**
  necrotic, 32–33
  streptococcal, **80–81**
Central nervous system
  mucormycosis of, 52
  toxoplasmosis of, **39–40**
Cephalosporins
  as *Hemophilus influenzae* meningitis treatment, 6
  ineffectiveness as *Pasteurella multocida* infection treatment, 59
  as pseudomembranous colitis treatment, 2
Cerebrospinal fluid, in amebic meningoencephalitis, 60,61
Chancre, syphilitic, 16, 17
Chancroid, **47–48**
Chest pain, pneumococcal pneumonia-related, 159, 160
Chest x-ray
  bilateral pulmonary opacities on, 112–113
  of chlamydial pneumonia, 145, 146
  lower lobe opacities on, 97, 98
  of measles, 184, 185
  of mycoplasmal pneumonia, 143
  of pneumococcal pneumonia, 159, 160, 161
  of right-sided staphylococcal endocarditis, 92, 93

Children
  arboviral encephalitis in, 36–37
  cerebral malaria in, 68
  erythema infectiosum in, 64–66
  streptococcal pharyngitis in, 86
Chills
  dysentery-related, 171
  malaria-related, 68, 135, 136, 137
  peritonitis-related, 158
Chlamydial infections
  endocarditis, 83,84
  gonorrhea-associated, 4
  lymphogranuloma venereum, 29
  pneumonia, **145–146**
  urethritis, 22, 23
Chloroquine, as malaria treatment, 68, 136, 137
Chronic ambulatory peritoneal dialysis, peritonitis associated with, **157–158**
Chronic obstructive pulmonary disease (COPD), 97–98, 160
Citrobacter freundii infection, 117
Clindamycin, as clostridial diarrhea risk factor, 2
Clostridial infections
  gas gangrene, **43–44**
  pseudomembranous colitis, **1–2**
Coccidiodomycosis, 180
Cold agglutinin titers
  in chlamydial pneumonia, 145, 146
  in mycoplasmal pneumonia, 143, 144, 146
Colitis
  Clostridium difficule-associated pseudomembranous, **1–2**
  strongyloidiasis-related, 91
Collagen vascular disease, syphilis serologic test results in, 79
Congestive heart failure, 149, 150
Conjunctival suffusion/conjunctivitis
  arboviral encepahlitis-related, 37
  Kawasaki disease-related, 166
  leptospirosis-related, 138, 139
  measles-related, 70, 71
  Rocky Mountain spotted fever-related, 114, 115
Constipation, enteric fever-related, 127
Coronary artery bypass patients
  drug fever in, **116–117**
  streptococcal leg cellulitis in, 81
Coronary artery disease, 146
Corticosteroids, as *Hemophilus influenzae* meningitis treatment, 6
Cough
  aspiration pneumonia-related, 31
  legionnaire's disease-related, 147, 148
  measles-related, 70, 71
  mycoplasmal pneumonia-related, 143, 144
  right-sided endocarditis-related, 92, 93
Coxiella burnetii, as endocarditis causal agent, 83, 84
Coxsackievirus infections
  hand-foot-mouth disease, 55
  meningitis, 163
Cramps, abdominal, 45, 46